Amazing Medicines The Drug Companies Don't Want You To Discover!

Amazing Medicines The Drug Companies

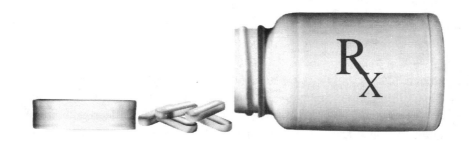

Don't Want You To Discover!

By
University Medical Research
Publishers

Tempe, Arizona 85281

Notice: This book is a reference volume and does not constitute medical advice. It should not be used as a manual for self treatment. The information herein was compiled to help you make informed choices about your health. The publishers cannot guarantee the safety or effectiveness of any drug, treatment or advice mentioned. We recommend in all cases that you should consult a licensed, professional health care provider before taking or discontinuing any medications or before treating yourself in any way.

Library of Congress Cataloging-in-Publication Data:

Amazing Medicines The Drug Companies Don't Want You Or Your Doctor To Discover/by the staff of University Medical Research Publishers.

Edited by: Staff

ISBN 0-9638714-0-4 hardcover.

1. Medicine, popular. 1.Staff 11. University Medical Research Publishers (Tempe, Arizona 85281)

10 9 8 7 6 5

Printed in the United States of America
University Medical Research Publishers
Tempe, Arizona 85281

CONTENTS

Carefully Tested!

You are about to learn some cold hard realities about the drug companies, their "alleged" watchdog—the Federal Drug Administration (FDA), the widespread greed of doctors and, most important, medicines that work for which you don't need a doctors prescription.

You'll also learn about a few prescription drugs not available in the U.S. that have proven to be sensational answers to certain problems and how to get them.

In the field of alternative medicine, you are exposed to a lot of stories about the benefits of certain vitamins, nutritional supplements, herbs, flavinoids and other organic extracts. Unfortunately, most of it is written by vitamin companies or herbalists who are touting their products and often stretch the truth.

Today we live in a scientific world where technology has reached a point that we can test the use of a medicine or nutritional supplement and carefully evaluate its effects in an unbiased way.

The Importance of Double Blind Studies!

The accepted method of evaluating a substance by scientists worldwide is called a "double blind" study. A scientist must eliminate the possibility of bias and the "placebo effect".

The placebo effect is simply the power of our minds to achieve what it believes will happen if a certain medicine is taken.

In a double blind study, the director does not have any contact with the patients being tested. Researchers handle the patients. The director makes up one group of pills (for example) that contain the ingredient being tested and an inert substance. He also makes up another batch of pills that look identical but contain only the inert substance. These are placebos.

The researchers are given packets of pills marked for a specific patient. They don't know whether the pills are placebos or the real thing. All patients are told that they are receiving something that should help them, which prevents the placebo effect from skewing the results. Also, it is less likely that the researcher can influence the results.

If the real ingredient shows substantially more positive results than the placebo and there are enough patients tested, the study will be considered statistically valid.

When the results are published in a scientific journal, other scientists around the world try to duplicate the results in another double blind study. If they can, then scientists in this field usually believe that the ingredient has value.

266 Double Blind Studies Are Covered!

In this book, our research team examined 266 research projects conducted by over 500 medical scientists worldwide. We eliminated all claims for non-prescription medicines and supplements where there was no scientific testing done. In most cases, we name the scientists and where the results were published so you can investigate further if you wish.

The purpose of this book is to make you aware of natural substances you can use not only to prevent illnesses and diseases, but also ones which cure or alleviate the disorder.

A portion of medical scientists believe that we can prevent many illnesses except where they are genetically caused. And every day, genetic researchers are discovering genes that cause certain diseases and ways to manipulate these genes to correct specific problems.

Health care in the future is certain to be mostly preventive maintenance or genetic correction instead of just trying to control the symptoms as doctors do today.

We are finally learning in a big way how to correct the causes not only the symptoms. Hippocrates would be proud!

—THE EDITORS.

The License To Legally Rip Off The Public!

The U.S. Patent Office describes a patentable item as one that is new, unique, not in existence prior to being created by the inventor and performs a useful purpose. Therefore something that exists in a plant, animal, earth or air is not patentable.

For example, salicylic acid which is found in the bark of poplar and willow trees, is commonly known as aspirin. It could not be patented when it was discovered. All vitamins and minerals exist in plants and animals, and, of course, can't be patented.

The big drug companies don't want to market anything for which they can't get a patent. The reason is that other companies could also make the product and the ensuing competition would cause the price and profit margins to be very low. That means that all patent protected drugs are essentially "designer chemicals", not natural substances.

So, a low profit margin on medicines from natural sources is the reason the drug companies don't want you or your doctor to know about those medicines!

Most Profitable Business In The World!

Chemical World, a business magazine that services the pharmaceutical or drug industry as well as other chemical users, recently reported that "The drug business is one of the most profitable industries in the world."

The reason is that the federal government gives the drug companies a monopoly on a newly patented drug for 17 years and they can charge any price they wish. No one can copy that drug or create a generic for 17 years.

On the surface that's fair because inventor's creativity should be protected. However, we're not discussing inventing a Polaroid camera. The Polaroid inventor had 17 competition free years to recoup his development costs and be rewarded with the profits from his creativity. But there is a difference between a product such as a camera, and a drug.

When the Polaroid camera was first sold it was so expensive that only upper income people could afford it. However, there is a common law in economics that states, "the more people who can afford your product, the more you will sell". Polaroid followed that law and steadily found ways to lower the price of the camera over the 17 years so more people could afford it. This was in spite of the fact that inflation caused labor and material costs to go up an average of 5% per year.

They Charge As Much As They Think You Can Afford!

Drug companies don't have to deal with this basic law of economics because patients are told by their doctors that they MUST have the drug. Therefore the drug companies charge as much as they think the market can bear.

The cost of manufacturing most drugs is minuscule compared to the price charged. The bottle, label and box often cost as much or more than the ingredients.

When questioned about their prices, the drug companies scream, "we spend $100 to $250 million developing and testing a drug before we market it. We have to amortize that cost into every bottle we sell."

On the surface that sounds like a legitimate argument except for some interesting questions. One, why are drug companies' net profits the highest of all industries? Two, why is it that European drug manufacturers, which have equal or even higher labor costs than the United States, spend an average of only $50 million per drug to develop and test it?

According to the annual statements of the large publicly traded drug companies, last year they spent about $8 billion on research and development of drugs. However, they also spent OVER $10 BILLION ON ADVERTISING! Of course, advertising cost is also amortized into the price of each drug.

Why Must A Prescription Drug Be Advertised?

This $10 billion expenditure indicates that advertising should be about 50% of a drug company's cost for the drug. After they add their profit margin and overhead to make a wholesale price, and pharmacies and hospitals double it again for their profit, a $5 cost of advertising becomes $20 to the patient.

But what we don't understand is why they must spend so much on advertising. The public can't buy their drugs without prescriptions. The costs of mailing an announcement and test results to doctors couldn't be more than a couple of dollars each or about $1 million per drug.

And at most there are less than 100 "new" drugs brought to market in even the most prolific years. So that amounts to $100 million to get the information to doctors in a year. Where do they spend the other $9.9 billion of their advertising expenses?

Well, we've found that a substantial portion of it goes to bribe doctors to prescribe each drug. Yes, they seriously bribe doctors! We'll give you the details in the next chapter.

How Drug Companies Create Patients For New Drugs!

The balance of their advertising is directed at the public, apparently to convince us that we have a medical problem which we didn't realize we had. Rarely does one of their "public service" ads mention a specific product because they would have to mention all the side effects. But if you go to the doctor for that medical problem, you can bet the only drug available is theirs.

The Public Health Information You Are Getting From The Media May Be Pure "Hype"!

Most of the time, their public relations experts create stories and send them to newspapers, magazines, TV and radio stations as "public service" or "educational" announcements. The drug companies cleverly avoid mentioning a product name, so the media immediately sends it out to the public as "news". The stories are described better as "scare the consumer" publicity campaigns.

These scare tactics definitely create a demand for the drugs. In fact, *The Wall Street Journal* quoted Jerry Jackson, the marketing chief for the drug company Merck, as saying, "We had to create a market as well as develop a drug." He was referring to Merck's new anti-cholesterol drug, LOVASTATIN.

Most Money Spent On Cholesterol Drugs!

Most people with high cholesterol can control it by changing their diet, but many people are lazy and would rather take a pill. Two of the highest dollar grossing prescription drugs are for cholesterol.

And it seems the cholesterol story changes every time you pick up the newspaper. First, it was that all cholesterol is bad. Then we had good and bad. The most recent one was that some of the good is bad. Next week we'll probably hear that some of the bad is good. Yet many scientists insist that the doctors are treating a symptom and not a cause.

Another very successful scare campaign was on high blood pressure. Literally hundreds of thousands feared they had a problem and visited their doctor who promptly gave them a new high blood pressure drug.

Although it may have helped a few people with extremely high blood pressure, mild pressure readings can usually be controlled with diet and lifestyle changes.

Talking Stomach Is Selling Ulcer Drugs!

You've probably seen the TV commercial with the animated stomach talking about ulcers. The drug company, SmithKline & French are responsible for the ad, and coincidently also make the ulcer drug, TAGAMET. Sales of this one drug last year was over $1 BILLION. Just mention heartburn or ulcers to your doctor. We bet that you'll walk away with a prescription for TAGAMET!

There has been an extensive ad campaign recently by the drug company, Merck, to "educate" men on the dangers of prostate disease. They manufacture the new prostate drug, PROSCAR.

But apparently, it is not doing too well. Most general practitioners will refer you to a urologist if they suspect that you have a prostate disorder. Much to Merck's dismay, the urologists are not writing many prescriptions for PROSCAR.

Urologists Would Rather Cut
Than Give Drugs!

A recent article in *Newsweek* stated, "The problem, it seems, is that urologists would rather do surgery than prescribe a drug that MIGHT CUT BACK ON THEIR BUSINESS" (our emphasis).

In this case, that disturbs us greatly because it has been proven that surgery is practically worthless. Even though PROSCAR isn't effective in many cases, it would be better for the patients than surgery. But we've found much better natural medicine for prostate problems which we'll detail for you in the chapter on this subject.

Some Drug Prices Rose 1843% In Only 10 Years!

In 1982, a standard package of children's vaccines was priced at $7.00. 10 years later, that same package averages $130.00! There's no difference in the contents, and the cost of producing those vaccines hasn't risen much above the cost of inflation—about 5% per year. 5% compounded for 10 years would only raise the price to about $10.30. Maybe someone at the drug company put their decimal in the wrong place!

Drug Cost 50% Less In European Countries!

In Europe, the prices of American made drugs average 50% less than they do in the United States. The reason is that the health insurers there, which are often the governments, just won't pay any more than that.

These drugs are made by the same manufacturers, contain the same ingredients and are produced in the same controlled conditions as in the United States.

Our Government Allows Drug Companies To Gouge Us!

The government has allowed the drug companies to grab us right where it hurts and wring every nickel out of us. Americans are charged more because health insurance and government Medicare/Medicaid programs pay for 80% of our prescription drugs. President and Mrs. Clinton could cut health care costs almost in half if they forced drug companies to sell their drugs at the same price as in as Europe and stopped them from spending $10 billion on bribes and advertising.

Life is sacred. Why shouldn't good health also be sacred? When you are in pain or your life is threatened, you'll pay anything for relief, and the drug companies know it. Is that fair and democratic? Is good health so much less sacred that the government should allow scheming profiteers to gouge us every step of the way to death?

Cheaper For Sheep Than People!

Dr. Charles Moertel, a cautious cancer reseacher at the Mayo Clinic, discovered that a deworming drug used for sheep, levamisole, could reduce the reoccurance of colon cancer in human.

Under a $11 million federal grant, Dr. Moertal tested it on 1300 colon cancer patients and proved that levamisole reduced reoccurance by 41% and the overall death rate by 33%. The government gave Johnson & Johnson approval to market it to humans (brand name, Ergamisol).

Shortly thereafter, Mrs. Annie Rhymes of Rockport, Illinois was operated on for colon cancer. Her doctor prescribed levamisole (Ergamisol) after her release from the hospital.

She was dumbstruck when her pharmacist said it would cost $200 for a month's prescription–especially since she knew that the same drug for sheep sold locally for $6.39.

An Over-The-Counter Drug Rip Off!

Sandoz Pharmaceuticals found a simple way to double its profits: water down the medicine by 50%, put it in the same size bottle and charge the same price!

According to *U.S. News & World Report*, attorneys general in 34 states accused Sandoz of doing exactly that with their TRIAMINIC Cold And Cough Medicine For Children. And they had the gall to call it, "New, Improved".

Sandoz has agreed to drop the "improved" from its label and give customers refunds or coupons for an additional bottle. Send the label or other proof of purchase to: Sandoz Consumer, Box 476, East Hanover, NJ 07936. Indicate whether you want cash or a coupon.

Orphan Drug Act Being Trickily Manipulated!

The Orphan Drug Act was enacted by Congress in 1983 to encourage drug companies to develop remedies for people who have rare diseases. The Act states that there must be less than 200,000 people with the disease.

Any pharmaceutical company that develops an orphan drug gets a tax credit for up to 50% of the development and marketing costs, plus a seven year monopoly on the drug if it is not patentable.

Government Gave Taxol To Squibb!

The Act was a great concept, but it has been totally abused by drug companies with our government's approval. For example, take TAXOL, the new drug for ovarian cancer that was found in the bark of the yew tree. Our government funded National Cancer Institute (NCI) spent $30 million developing and proving that TAXOL works. It was then "given" to Squibb Company to finish the FDA required testing and market it.

Even though Squibb had very little expense in bring TAXOL to cancer patients, the charge for it ranges from $4,000.00 to $6,000.00 per year for each patient according to the *New York Times*. If that isn't patient exploitation, we don't know what is.

Officials of Ralph Nader's Center For Study of Responsive Law says that NCI paid another drug company only 12% of Squibb's wholesale price to make the initial supplies of TAXOL for testing. The Orphan Drug Act does not control what the drug companies charge!

New studies by NCI show that TAXOL also works on six other malignancies, including lung and breast cancer, which together afflict over 160,000 yearly. It is also being tested on 18 other cancers with high hopes. TAXOL will be a bonanza for Squibb even without the benefits of the Orphan Drug Act—yet the FDA is leaving it under the Act.

$300,000 A Year For One Prescription!

Another orphan, CEREDASE, the drug for Gaucher's Disease, costs some patients, Medicare or health insurance companies over $300,000 a year per patient.

AZT, the AIDS drug, was also developed by government scientists with your tax dollars. Burroughs-Welcome was given the exclusive under the Orphan Act and began charging patients $10,000.00 a year each. Only after intense pressure by political activists, they dropped the price to $6,400.00.

Slicing The Salami!

Drug companies also use the trick of slicing up the market for a drug to qualify for the Orphan Act. The slang for the trick in the industry is "slicing the salami".

Here's how it is done. Let's assume a company creates a drug for asthma but applies under the Act as a treatment for the rare steriod dependent asthma. Less than 200,000 people have this rare disease. Yet now the drug company has a drug protected and benefited by the Act but will probably sell it to all 10 million asthma sufferers.

According to *The Wall Street Journal*, Biogen, Inc., developed the drug "r-IFN-beta". They applied and received Orphan privileges as a treatment for metastic renal cell carcinoma. Three months later, the same drug company applied and received Orphan Act privileges for using it to treat cutaneous malignant melanoma.

And then after two weeks, the company applied for and received Orphan Act status for treating cutaneous T-cell melanoma. But that wasn't enough. Shortly thereafter, the FDA approved Biogen's Orphan application for treating some AIDS related conditions.

Biogen has a market of nearly a million patients for a drug that it split into five applications; yet the FDA looks the other way. This is a case of severe abuse of the Act, and taxpayers are footing the bill.

Congress Quietly Changed The Act To Benefit Drug Companies!

When the Act was first written in 1983, it required drug companies to show that the potential market was too small to be profitable. In 1984, due to the tremendous power and money of the drug company lobbyists, the Act was quietly amended, leaving out that requirement. Not only do we have crooked drug companies, but our elected politicians are their co-conspirators!

2

United State Senate Hearing On Drug Company Fraud And Bribery!

The scare publicity campaigns by drug companies are a more recent scheme to market drugs. The old standby method is to "encourage" or bribe doctors into prescribing certain drugs. There are about a dozen major drug companies and many smaller ones that make generics, so bribery can be quite lucrative for doctors.

Much of this chapter has been excerpted from the transcript of a Senate hearing before the Senate Committee On Labor And Human Resources chaired by Senator Edward Kennedy. The primary testimony is by Dr. Sidney Wolfe, M.D., director of the Public Citizens Health Research Group, a non-profit watchdog of the drug industry.

Dr. Wolfe obtained many of his leads for the information he gave at the hearing from a Doctor Bribing Hotline where doctors, doctors' office personnel, drug company employees and others report unethical and illegal behavior of the drug companies.

Free $35,000.00 Doctor's Office Computer System!

The most outrageous case of bribery that Dr. Wolfe found was executed by a company called Physicians Computer Network (PCN). This company was really a front organization for the 10 largest drug companies.

PCN gave doctors a big, elaborate "practice management" software and hardware package that computerizes details on every patient, the diagnosis of their ills, the drugs prescribed and does billing and other bookkeeping chores.

There were two conditions necessary to receive this equipment: one, allow PCN to hook it to a phone modem so they can access the information anytime (except for name and address of the patient); and two, the doctor must watch 32 ads a month that appear on this computer system and answer one clinically oriented question per ad. Now that's very cheap conditions for a $35,000.00 system—about 32 minutes of the doctor's time per month.

How Do The Drug Companies Benefit?

First, they get incredibly accurate and valuable marketing information about patients which they could NOT get else where which they use probably, to fuel for the scare campaigns and to convince other doctors to prescribe their drugs.

Second, they get to view the doctor's prescribing habits. That information is passed on to each drug company's "detail persons". They are actually sales people who call on doctors, giving them free samples and promoting certain drugs. Obviously, the sales person will corner the doctor asking why he or she is prescribing a competitor's drug.

Third, and most important, the drug companies have a captive audience with the 32 ads that the doctor must watch in order to answer a question about each. A psychologist told us that this is a highly clever and effective way to advertise because the doctor must concentrate on each ad to answer the question. By doing that, the information will probably stay in the doctor's memory. When those symptoms appear in a patient, the doctor is very likely to prescribe the drug he saw on the computer ad.

This information has been turned over to the Human Health Services (HHS) Inspector General for possibly bringing bribery action against the drug companies.

$1,200.00 Cash For Prescribing Expensive Antibiotics!

Sales people from the drug company, Roche, contacted doctors asking them to participate in a "clinical study" for their synthetic variant of penicillin called ROCEPHIN.

The salesperson virtually dictated a letter to the doctor's secretary that was to be sent by the doctor to Roche requesting money for the "study". Roche responded by immediately sending the doctor a letter of acceptance with a check for $600.00 stating that another $600.00 would be sent when the study was finished.

All the doctor had to do was record the age, diagnosis, antibiotic sensitivity, dose and duration of therapy using ROCEPHIN of 20 hospitalized patients. It may seem like a lot to do, but it required only four minutes per patient. That's 80 minutes of work for which the doctor received $1,200.00—equivalent to $900.00 per hour.

How Did The Drug Company Make Out On This "Study"?

The wholesale prices of drugs are listed in a book for pharmacists called the Redbook. From 1990 Redbook prices, Dr. Wolfe calculated that two grams of ROCEPHIN given to 20 patients for ten days would result in gross wholesale revenues of $11,400. $1,200 in promotional costs to generate $11,400 in sales is quite a bargain.

But it is no bargain for the patients, Medicare and the health insurance companies. The hospital will double the wholesale price and bill the patients for $22,800. That's about $15,000 higher than the cost of generic penicillin. ROCEPHIN is just a synthetic version of penicillin.

Roche is hiding behind its very thin veil of "alleged research". What will happen? Well, now that it has been reported to HHS, and they've started an investigation; Roche will probably drop the program and start a different one.

1000 Frequent Flier Miles For Every Prescription Written!

The drug company, Wyeth-Ayerst created a program to protect the sales of its INDERAL, a hypertension drug which had just run out of its 17 years of patent protection.

In a cooperative deal with American Airlines, Wyeth offered doctors 1,000 frequent flier miles for every prescription of INDERAL written. All the doctor had to do was fill out a simple form which required a few words about the patient's condition and what drug INDERAL replaced.

The doctor has to write ONLY 50 prescriptions to be rewarded with a free ticket ANYWHERE in the United States. It's possible that some doctors write that many hypertension drug prescriptions in a week!

American Airlines would not reveal how many doctors had flown at Wyeth's expense, but an American Airlines spokesman did say, "It was a very successful program from our standpoint."

A few thousand passengers probably wouldn't be significant, so we bet that literally tens of thousands of doctors took the bribe.

Obviously the drug companies know that there are a lot of unethical doctors who will go for these bribes—otherwise they wouldn't keep using these programs.

Only One State Has A Law Against Doctor Bribery!

Massachusetts is the only state that has a law against doctor bribery by drug companies, but it applies ONLY when Medicaid paid for the drug. That leaves individuals and health insurance companies out in the cold.

In 1989, Massachusetts launched a criminal investigation of Wyeth Ayerst which later culminated in the following statement:

> The pharmaceutical company, Wyeth Ayerst, which promoted the use of a new heart drug by offering Massachusetts physicians free airline tickets, diagnostic equipment and medical books will pay the Commonwealth of Massachusetts $195,000.00 and cease its promotional program as part of an agreement reached today with Attorney General James M. Shannon.

"This office is increasingly concerned with marketing practices of pharmaceutical companies which provide gifts and other incentives designed to influence physicians in prescribing drugs—a practice that violates the state's Medicaid False Claims Act," Shannon said. "It is important that medical decisions be made solely on the best interests of the patient and not on the basis of inducements offered by drug companies."

Also there is a federal law that prohibits bribery, but only where Medicare or Medicaid payments are involved. Even the federal government doesn't think the rest of us are important.

HHS claimed they were investigating this case, but no publicly announced results were found! We wonder why?

A Variation On Green Stamps
For Writing Prescriptions!

Connaught Laboratories was caught by HHS giving doctors "points" redeemable in merchandise for every vaccine package that they prescribed. The merchandise included VCRs, video cameras, computers, software, TVs, medical equipment and medical education programs.

HHS Inspector General Richard Kusserow wrote, "This program functions like the supermarket green stamp programs of the past."

Connaught was neither indicted nor sued. They claimed no Medicare or Medicaid funds were involved but agreed to discontinue the program. Not even a slap on the wrist. It's amazing what the drug companies can get away with.

$100 Bribe To Get Doctors To Prescribe
A Dangerous Drug!

Dr. Ken Arndt, a dermatology professor at Harvard, received a letter from Sandoz regarding the use of SANDIMMUNE, its immune suppression drug. The FDA had approved it ONLY for preventing organ rejection in people receiving kidney transplants.

The purpose of the letter was to get Dr. Arndt to read a two page report on the use of SANDIMMUNE to treat psoriasis. He was promised $100.00 if he would answer some questions afterwards.

Dr. Ardnt was outraged by this as it appeared to be a blatant bribery campaign to get doctors to prescribe the drug for an UNAPPROVED purpose.
Dr. Ardnt pointed out that a recent article in the *British Journal of Dermatology* stated that 46% of people being treated with this drug for psoriasis had to discontinue because of serious side effects.

There are no reports of Sandoz being reprimanded for bribery. Why is the federal government looking the other way?

Wining, Dining And Pocket Lining!

Regularly doctors are being paid $100.00 to $200.00 plus a gourmet dinner with expensive wines at exclusive, pricey hotels to listen to lectures on the benefits of new drugs. The drug companies get around any bribery complaints by calling the payments "honorariums" or "consulting fees".

How Successful Are These Bribes?

An article in the drug promotion magazine, *Medical Marketing And Media*, said the increasingly wide-spread practice of promotional dinners will be attended by 175,000 to 180,000 doctors this year (1990).

A promotional dinner expert commenting on the ultimate measure of success of these events (increased prescription sales) said, "Every promotional dinner doesn't result in a marked increase in the sales curve. They fail 15% to 20% of the time."

Well, in the general marketing world an 80% to 85% success ratio is considered almost unbelievably successful. If a salesperson could sell 8 out 10 prospects approached, he or she would be considered the greatest salesperson in the world.

Doctor Bribing Hotline!

If you are ever in a position to observe or obtain knowledge of other bribery by drug companies, please report it to the Hotline, 202-872-0320. Ask for Dr. Sidney Wolfe. Let's keep up the pressure on this. Maybe something will happen.

Death By Doctor Error Or Bribery?

A Harvard study reported that over 10,000 people died in one year in New York City hospitals due to doctors' mistakes or malpractice. By extrapolating that figure nationwide, we estimate that 186,000 people die across the country from doctors misprescribing drugs or practicing medicine poorly. Doctors even have a fancy word for it. They say, "The person died of 'iatrogenic' causes!"

Perhaps many of those people died because doctors prescribed the wrong drugs due to the influence of getting a drug company bribe.

If a judge gets caught accepting a bribe, usually he or she will get prison time and the total loss of reputation and career. But the decision which was influenced by the bribe will only cost the loser some money or maybe time in jail. Rarely does it result in death.

Yet, if a drug company bribes a doctor, and he or she, due to greed, kills someone with the wrong prescription, nothing happens to either the doctor or the drug company. Isn't it time we did something about this awful situation?

Drug Companies Lie To Doctors!

Sometimes the doctor can't be blamed for misprescribing drugs. For example, the FDA approved the drug DIPENTUM for use only in adults to help them maintain remission of ulcerative colitis. Kabi Pharmacia, Inc., the manufacturer, sent its representatives to doctors claiming CHILDREN COULD USE IT, that it was the best choice for all stages of active ulcerative colitis; and that it was superior to SULVASALAZINE, the generic drug for this disease.

Apparently none of these claims were proven and accepted by the FDA. *The Wall Street Journal* reported that a consent decree signed by Kabi and filed in Federal Court demands the company stop making unproven claims to doctors and spend $300,000.00 to advertise that DIPENTUM's only use was the original one approved by the FDA.

Apparently this happens all the time. FDA Commissioner Dr. David Kessler said, "As a physician, I think we would be burying our head in sand to assume that this is an isolated instance. The company's goal was to increase sales AT THE EXPENSE OF PATIENT CARE (our emphasis)."

Pervasive Mischief In
The Drug Industry!

A psychiatrist charged the drug company Upjohn with falsifying scientific evidence regarding the safety of their sleeping pill, HALCION. The British Department Of Health banned sales of the drug in England while our government conducted an investigation. Upjohn countered with denials and a libel suit against the psychiatrist. HALCION is still on the market in the United States.

In 1988 the FDA investigated Hoffman-La Roche for an alleged coverup of the deadly effects of its anesthetic, VERSED, which had been tied to 40 deaths from respiratory failure. A congressional subcommittee also investigated, but the drug is still on the market.

Pfizer has set up a $500 million fund for problems from its now discontinued artificial heart valves. They have a tendency to crack inside the body killing the person according to a story in *Time Magazine*.

The most recent and biggest story is about Dow Corning Wright who is accused of failing to report that its silicone gel breast implants were associated with severe side effects such as rheumatoid arthritis and lupus. Between 1 and 2 million women have implants made by Dow and other manufacturers.

Breast Implant Problems Hidden
In Dow Memos!

Dr. Norman Anderson, one of the FDA's advisory panel members, said that he was amazed when he read dozens of documents from a breast implant liability suit. Apparently 17 Dow internal memos dating back to the mid-1970s revealed numerous problems with the implants.

Dow had previously assured the FDA that they had disclosed all relevent details about the implants. However, Dr. Anderson concluded that the memos leave "...little doubt of Dow's misrepresentation of the facts." The FDA declared a moratorium on sales of the implants while it studies the problem.

Yes, "studies" the problem. In our minds, this was a criminal act. We've seen people go to jail for a lot less. It's about time that the government started putting some drug company executives in jail. That might stop some of this rampant corruption.

The drug company Bolar allegedly forged documents seeking FDA approval of DYAZIDE, its generic high blood pressure pill. Also, the pill was found to be defective. Bolar was fined $10 million and its pills pulled from the market. Bolar's top executive, Robert Shulman, went to jail.

Drug Company Substitutes Proven Drug For Its Test Results!

Generic drug manufacturers must prove to the FDA that their drug performs the same as the formerly patent protected drug. The research director of Vitane Pharmaceuticals ordered a proven brand name drug to be substituted for their generic version of the drug in the required equivalency tests.

He also forged the initials of employees on test batches and raised the size of the test batches in reports to the FDA, according to a story in the *Washington Post*.

The company sold more than $11 million of the drug, triamterene hydrochlorothiazide, before the government recalled it.

20 executives of the company have been convicted or pleaded guilty to charges of fraud, racketeering and obstruction of justice. The company was fined $2 million and now is in bankruptcy.

Generic drug companies are usually very small in comparison to the top ten companies. Vitane would be a grain of sand next to a boulder if compared to the top ten. Why is it that the FDA viciously attacks the little companies and not the big boys? We suspect the big ones have too much political power.

10th Generic Drug Company To Plead Guilty In Three Years!

Vitane was the tenth drug company to plead guilty to fraud and mis-representation in the last three years. U.S. District Judge John Hargrove said, "There is virtually no testing of some products...and they are thrown out into the market."

FDA Employees Taking Bribes!

During the investigation of those 10 companies, detectives discovered that five key employees of the FDA had taken bribes from the drug companies to speed up the approval of their applications for new drugs.

Get A Big Grant For A Positive Story!

Last year allegations arose regarding research grants by drug companies to prominent scientists. It seems the grants were conditioned on the scientists writing positive papers on new drugs about to be marketed—and those papers being published in a major medical journal.

The grants ranged as high as $50,000.00 and involved several scientists and drug companies. Sources claim papers were actually published; which, of course, influenced perhaps hundreds of thousands of doctors to prescribe the drugs.

No intense investigation was done because both the scientists and the drug companies denied any collusion. We think the investigators were pretty naive to expect either party to admit to something so devastating to careers of the scientists and the profits of the companies.

Drug Companies Test New Drugs Under An "Honor System"!

When drug companies test a new drug, they don't have to submit the raw data to the FDA. The FDA relies on the companies' own analyses and conclusions.

Often it takes 10 years from creation through testing until a drug comes to the market. Drug companies claim the cost ranges from $50 million to $250 million per drug.

Let's say your drug company has spent $200 million, and it discovers some problems with the drug. A $200 million investment is a mighty big incentive to downplay the problems. *Time Magazine* quoted Robert Temple, chief of the FDA's Office of Drug Evaluation, as saying: "They definitely have rose colored glasses!"

The FDA makes big promises of changes in the system. FDA chief Robert Kessler told the press, "The honor system is out the window..." That sounds great, but Washington observers say that the FDA has neither the staff nor subpoena powers to discover problems before it is too late.

Just how a profit driven system can be expected to operate on honor and trust is beyond us. Yet every sick person's life is depending on it!

Drug Companies Won't Release Safety Trial Results!

In England, the British Parliment has proposed the Medicines Information Bill. This bill, if passed, would provide the public with a full report on the safety trials of each drug. British drug companies, several of which are owned by American drug companies, are fighting it vehemently with the most suspicious defense.

They claim it would eliminate healthy competition between drug companies. Maybe that's exactly what we need—less competition and more human concern!

Adverse Reactions In 4 Point Greek!

Occasionally with a prescription drug you get a leaflet in the package that describes possible side effects of the drug. If you have a powerful magnifying glass, possibly you can read the tiny, crammed together 4 point type (that's one third the size of the type on this page), but understanding the language requires a doctorate degree in biology, chemistry or medicine.

Dorothy Smith, president of the Consumer Health Information Service, says, "97% of the material on drugs written for patients cannot be understood by the average consumer."

People over 60 are affected more than anyone because they take 59% of all the prescriptions. Vision gets poorer the older they get and many have less than a high school education.

Why are the drug companies hiding the truth about drugs? Is it so bad that no one would risk taking the drug? Or is it that they are not concerned about the patient's well being? It's pretty obvious to us that they don't care and want to hide any problems.

Doctors Don't Know That Drug Side Effects On Elderly People Are Worse!

Most doctors are not aware that the dosage of many drugs should be much lower for elderly people. 70% of doctors treating Medicare patients flunked an exam concerning their knowledge of prescribing to older adults.

Also certain combinations of drugs are dangerous such as taking WARFARIN, a blood thinning agent, while taking aspirin. It can lead to fatal bleeding in some elderly people.

The average elderly person takes four prescription drugs and two nonprescription substances. Often they experience side effects caused by the combination, but usually write it off as just another affliction of old age.

Drug companies are not required to make any tests specifically on elderly people to see if the dosage should be modified. The big pussycat FDA folks said they issued a guideline in March 1993 that STRONGLY URGES drug manufacturers to evaluate the effects on elderly people and print the information on an enclosure to go with the drug. If they don't have any information that would have to be stated.

Well, whoop-tee-do! Why doesn't the FDA just whip them with a wet noodle? It would have about the same effect. We thought federal regulatory agencies made rules and regulations, not strongly worded urges!

Some Drugs Destroy Vital Nutrients!

Many drugs block vital nutrient uptake, according to a USDA financed study at the Human Nutrition Research Center On Aging at Tufts University. The more drugs you take and the longer you take them increases the risk of nutritional side effects.

Deficiency in a nutrient can cause other illnesses which may force you to go to the doctor again. Very few doctors have any education in nutrition, so they'll try to find another prescription drug in their kit for your problem. That's like pouring gasoline on an out-of-control fire!

Dr. Earl Mindell's *Vitamin Bible* lists 64 prescription and non-prescription drugs or medicines that rob your body of vital nutrients, such as: aspirin removes Vitamin C, B and folic acid; cortisone and prednisone steal zinc; laxatives and antacids deplete Vitamins A, D, E & K; and diuretics destroy potassium. Dr. Mindell's book is available in most book stores and is a worthy addition to any home library.

Adverse Reactions To Drugs!

According to the government's General Accounting Office (GAO), a study found that more than half of the prescription drugs approved by the FDA between 1976 and 1985 caused serious side effects. They were either pulled from the market or relabeled with warnings.

An FDA spokesman claimed the study was "alarmist and inaccurate"! The GAO accountants just compiled hard statistics and were less likely to lie than the FDA, which was protecting its territory.

Many of the side effects resulted in hospitalizations, permanent disability and death, according to the GAO report. A Public Citizen Health Research Group newsletter reported that 22% of older patients given three or more prescriptions upon release from hospitals had prescription errors that were potentially serious or life threatening.

With an estimated 186,000 people dying every year from iatrogenic causes (medically caused reasons), it is believed that a substantial portion were drug induced. According to published studies and the Public Citizen Research Group (PCRG), 119 out of 364 most commonly prescribed drugs for old people should not be used because safer alternatives are available and effective.

Every year 659,000 older adults have to be hospitalized due to drug side effects. Close to another 9 million suffer at home from these adverse drug reactions.

29 Drugs May Give You Parkinson's Disease!

This will shock you but it is true! Imagine taking a drug, and it causes the terrible, dehabilitating Parkinson's Disease. Well, over 61,000 people experienced that last year! There are actually 29 drugs on the market that can cause Parkinson's.

There are another 65 that can cause you to go crazy—dementia! PCHR says there are:

- 86 drugs that cause depression;
- 105 that cause hallucinations;
- 46 that can make you fall and probably break bones;
- 22 that can cause auto accidents;
- 119 that cause sexual problems;
- 88 that cause constipation;
- and 18 that will keep you from sleeping well!

If You Must Take Prescription Drugs...

There's a book that may give you some protection. PCHR, a non-profit association, has published a book, "Worst Pills/Best Pills II" by Dr. Sidney Wolfe. If offers the plain truth in understandable English about 346 drugs most commonly prescribed to older adults. It includes 70 of the newest, most promoted ones such as PROZAC, MEVACOR, CIPRO, PEP-CID and BuSPAR.

Dr. Wolfe and other experts warn about 119 of these drugs which they feel you shouldn't use, and what to use as safe, effective alternatives. The book is only $12.00 and has 722 pages.

Write to:
Public Citizen
2000 P. Street NW, Dept. AM
Washington, DC 20036

There's no shipping charge in the United States, but people in Canada and overseas must add $6.00.

3

FDA's Gestapo Tactics Against Vitamins!

On the suggestions from the FDA, state health inspectors in Texas last year raided health food and vitamin stores throughout the state and confiscated thousands of products. Shoppers were astounded as the inspectors took vitamin C, aloe vera products and herbal teas from the shelves.

Worst yet, in Kent, Washington, 16 bullet proof vested FDA agents brandishing guns burst into the Tahoma Clinic commanding the employees to "freeze".

The agents took all of Dr. Jonathon Wright's medical equipment (worth over $100,000.00), patients' records and his inventory of vitamins. Also they arrested the doctor.

The FDA claimed Dr. Wright was making illegal drugs and injecting them into patients. The "illegal drugs" were vitamins. Alex Straus, director of Citizens For Health, said, "For God's sake, we're talking about vitamin C and B_{12} shots!"

Like Rodney King Situation, Patient Films Attack!

Fortunately a patient in the waiting room had his video camera with him and recorded the whole fiasco. It was broadcast on news programs nationally.

The biggest newspaper in the area, the *Seattle Post*, warned in an editorial, "If there is any plausible excuse for the Gestapo-like tactics used in the raid of Dr. Wright's clinic, it better be forthcoming and fast!"

FDA Says Mixing Vitamins Is Illegal?

The FDA says its actions were "grounded in hard science and law".

Since when is mixing vitamins illegal? You can buy multi-vitamins everywhere! Also when was a law enacted that says doctors CANNOT inject vitamin B_{12} and other vitamins? Most doctors give B_{12} shots!

And now a year later, the FDA has not prosecuted or imposed criminal penalties in any of its raids. Yet they have not returned Dr. Wright's equipment, records or inventory—essentially putting the man out of business! We called the Texas state health inspectors office, and no one seemed to know whether they had returned the health food stores' merchandise.

What we're even more appalled at is the way government cops (city, county, state and federal) REGULARLY love to pretend to be Rambo or SWAT teams. They must love to dress up in their "shoot-`em-up" outfits! Why does it require a big powerful government agency to use 16 burly cops in bullet proof vests with guns drawn to serve a search warrant on a little doctor and three young female employees?

FDA Treated Them Like Columbian Drug Lords!

Neither the doctor nor any of his employees had arrest records. None of them even had a gun registered in their names. If a single government cop comes to most law abiding people's homes or businesses with a search warrant, do they pull out guns and try to shoot the cop? No! It's simply a case of cops and government out of control.

Fortunately the FDA Gestapo team drew tremendous heat from the public. Within 24 hours, over 2000 letters were sent to President Bush and hundreds more went to the FDA. Numerous non-profit citizens' groups were formed to assault Congress with their displeasure and rage.

Why is it a government agency that is supposed to protect our health allows big drug companies to get away with all kinds of fraud and chicanery, yet sticks guns in the faces of people taking and selling vitamins?

Few Medical Schools Teach Nutrition!

Most of the powerful executives at the FDA are doctors. Yet 102 out of 127 major medical schools DO NOT have courses on nutrition and vitamins. Just where do these doctors get their "superior" knowledge that vitamins don't have any effect on people? In fact, that is what most older doctors will say if you ask them if you should take vitamins.

This totally violates medical precedents set down all the way back to the 14th century when doctors discovered that sailors at sea for long periods without vegetables or fruits got scurvy—a Vitamin C deficiency!

Vitamin Deficiency Causes Many Illnesses!

The deficiency of practically any vitamin can and does cause illness or disease. Did the FDA forget that it polices the "RDA"—the MINIMUM daily requirement of vitamins and minerals everyone needs to maintain their health?

According to Dr. Earl Mindell, the author of the most comprehensive book on vitamins, minerals and nutrients, *The Vitamin Bible*, this is a partial list of the illnesses caused by deficiencies in some vitamins:

A Deficiency of	Causes
Vitamin A	Night blindness
Vitamin B_1	Beriberi, a nerve disorder
Vitamin B_2	Skin eruptions
Vitamin C	Nosebleeds & scurvy
Vitamin B_6	Anemia & dermatitis
Vitamin B_{12}	Anemia & neurological disorders
Vitamin B_5	Hypoglycemia & ulcers
Vitamin B	Pellagra & dermatitis
Vitamin D	Rickets & tooth decay
Vitamin E	Muscle degeneration & anemia

4

The No. 1 Reason For Becoming A Doctor— Money!

A survey of medical students revealed that 83% wanted to become doctors because of the big money they would earn! Did you really think people would go through years of tough medical school studies JUST to help sick people?

The average medical doctor in the United States earns in excess of $300,000 per year if they have their own practice. The top 20% earn over $1 million. Those that have doctors working for them (and heart surgeons) often earn over $3 million per year.

It's easy to see how heart surgeons make so much money when you look at the cost of open heart or bypass surgery. The price of that procedure ranges from $30,000.00 to $50,000.00. For a half day's work, the head surgeon will take home $15,000.00 to $25,000.00. The balance goes to the anesthesiologist, assisting surgeon and the hospital.

If the doctor averages just three a week, he or she will gross $3.9 million for the year with a month vacation. We would say that that kind of money is a pretty good incentive to go to medical school.

A Quick Way To Tell
If Your Doctor Is Greedy!

Many doctors make patients wait anywhere from 30 minutes to three hours before they see them—and then with no apology. In the normal business world, no one would make you wait for more than 30 minutes for a scheduled appointment. And then if it was more than 15 minutes, you'd get a very serious apology for being made to wait.

If you go into any retail business to spend money and are made to wait for more than a few minutes, most people would walk out and go to competitive store where their business will be appreciated.

Why Are Doctors Different?

Doctors found out long ago that they could get away with it because people are resistant to changing doctors. No matter how inconsiderate the doctor is of the patients' time, they still go back!

The doctors also found that about 5% of patients cancel their appointments at the last minute or don't show. Therefore doctors overbook patients to take up the slack.

Everyone gets delayed once in a while for unexpected reasons, and doctors are no different. But have you ever walked into a doctor's office in a major city at the exact time of your appointment and been immediately taken in to see the doctor?

They're Totally Inconsiderate Of You!

We took a survey of our office staff, and EVERYONE said that they have to wait every time they go to their doctor's office. The only exception was dentists. Many people said that they usually don't have to wait very long for their dentists.

So, if a doctor usually runs late everyday, why doesn't he or she book less appointments? Obviously they have no concern that you have to waste your valuable time sitting there reading old magazines.

What they are really concerned about is jamming as many patients into their schedule as possible in order to make as much money as they can.

An Easy $1.2 Million Profit Per Year!

Some doctors see as many as 12 patients per hour. With an average doctor's visit in most major cities running about $60.00, that's $720.00 per hour. In 8 hours they have grossed $5,760.00 less rent, utilities and office help. If the doctor does that five days a week, 48 weeks a year, he or she will take home about $1,200,000.00 annually.

If all the working adults in this country only go to their doctor once per year during normal working hours, and they wait an average of one hour; that's 183,000,000 work hours that Americans lost if on an hourly wage—or businesses lost on salaried employees. At only $10.00 an hour, doctors cost us almost $2 billion in lost wages.

How Many Doctors Are Unethical?

According to the drug promotion magazine, *Medical Marketing and Media*, 175,000 to 180,000 doctors accepted the $100.00 to $200.00 plus fine wine and gourmet food to listen to a pitch on a new drug—a clearly unethical practice.

There are no figures accessible on how many participated in drug company inducements to write certain prescriptions such as the frequent flier, points for merchandise, free computers, phony research study programs and etc.

There's a general attitude among the people in this country that it is all right to rip off insurance companies whenever given the chance. Doctors are probably no different. And there are no figures available on how many doctors overbill insurance companies and charge them for unnecessary lab tests, X-rays and etc.

Out of the 552,000 members of the American Medical Association (AMA), we're betting the same 83% who went into doctoring for money are unethical in some aspect of their practice.

A Clever And Profitable Reaction To Malpractice Insurance Rate Increases!

In the 1970s, insurance companies experienced a big surge in malpractice claims, so they dramatically increased their insurance rates to doctors. The outcry was enormous. Everytime you turned on TV or picked up a paper, doctors were claiming the increase would put them out of business or raise medical costs by 50%.

Of course, doctors are not dummies. They went to their attorneys to find out how they could avoid malpractice claims. Doctors with few or no claims were paying much lower insurance fees.

The attorneys said that there was a simple answer. Give the patients every kind of lab test, X-ray and other tests even remotely related to the patients' problems. This procedure would certainly cover the doctor in case something unusual popped up that could cause a claim.

Also, the attorneys and insurance companies made up a form for each patient to sign. That form, which goes under many different titles, essentially takes away the patient's rights to a jury trial and forces all malpractice claims into the hands of an arbitrator. Arbitrators rarely ever give high awards, especially million dollar ones, even where malpractice is clearly proven.

The attorneys also suggested that since the doctors would be conducting a high volume of medical tests, they could support their own laboratories and medical testing equipment. By doing that the doctors could double or triple their income.

Unethical For Doctors To Own
Related Businesses!

Up until the 1950s, the AMA considered it unethical for a doctor to own or have even an interest in laboratories, pharmacies, hospitals, clinics or drug companies (if they deal directly with patients).

It was called "double dipping" because the doctor would be making a profit from something he was prescribing. The AMA apparently felt that a greedy doctor could easily abuse that system with unnecessary tests, prescriptions, hospitalizations and etc.

However in the fifties, the AMA doctors voted out the old system and allowed themselves to own all sorts of businesses whose customers or patients could be generated from their practices.

The idea caught on slowly, probably because most doctors had been brought up with a more idealistic and ethical attitude toward medicine. But during the malpractice scare of the seventies, lawyers convinced many doctors that it was the thing to do. Of course, realizing they could double or triple their income was no small incentive either.

40% Of Doctors Own Labs Or
Treatment Facilities!

According to a survey by *Health Alert Newsletter*, doctors in Miami own 93% of all diagnostic MRI centers. However, in Baltimore, for some unknown reason, very few are owned by doctors. Would you want to take a guess at which doctors prescribed more $800.00 MRI scans? You're right. The Miami doctors scored twice as high as those in Baltimore!

The University of Arizona conducted a study of 65,000 patients. They found that doctors who had the MRI equipment in their offices conducted four times as many scans as doctors who referred patients elsewhere.

Over 40% of doctors own labs or treatment facilities. A study of a portion of those doctors showed that the doctors' labs did TWICE AS MANY TESTS PER PATIENT as independent labs—double dipping to the extreme.

But the independents are sacrosanct either. National Health Laboratories, Inc., in California was alleged caught in a fraudulent lab tests claims scheme. They agreed to return $111 MILLION to Medicare/Medicaid according to a story in *Playboy Magazine*.

Seminar For Bill Padding!

There are seminars that doctors pay to attend where they learn "creative billing". They are taught tricks of padding bills to get even more money out of your health insurance company. A story about this phenomenon appeared in the November 25, 1991 issue of *Time Magazine*.

Who pays for these padded bills and superfluous tests that are making doctors even more wealthy? Either you or your doctor pays higher insurance premiums. If employers pay more, then they must raise the price of their products or services to cover these additional costs. So even if you don't pay for health insurance directly, you pay for it with the higher prices of things you buy. Do doctors really deserve the tremendous amounts of money they get?

Overprescribing Drugs!

The *Washington Post* reported that Lurlyne Tompkins, 78, took nine drugs everyday: four pain medications, a thyroid drug, an ulcer drug, a diabetes drug, a high blood pressure drug and one for vascular problems. Her son discovered that often she didn't know whether it was day or night.

He took her and her basket of drugs to the Geriatric Assessment Center at John Hopkins Medical Institute. They found Mrs. Tompkins was taking several drugs she did not need and reduced the dosages of the ones she needed. Amy Goldstein, staff writer for the Washington Post wrote, "Mrs. Tompkins case is not rare...(it's) a common phenomena among elderly people."

Often elderly people have several doctors. Almost 40% of those over 65 take five prescription drugs daily. Another 19% take at least seven drugs, according to a study done by the National Council on Patient Information And Education.

Mixing Prescription Drugs Is Dangerous!

Mixing drugs can cause all sorts of problems—many of which are often unpredictable. The common reactions are diminished mental ability, dizziness, memory loss and bladder problems.

If you combine a high blood pressure drug with Valium, you may have severe mental problems. Arthritis drugs often react with coffee or alcohol to damage the stomach. Diuretics combined with heart medications multiplies the effect of each drug, which can be dangerous.

Even aspirin taken with blood thinning drugs can cause internal bleeding. Eye drops for glaucoma can cancel the benefits of diabetes and asthma drugs.

Doctors Should Ask!

Clearly it is the doctor's responsibility to ask patients what drugs they are already taking. However, you can't depend on them to ask or to know what is dangerous to mix. However, in any case, tell the doctor what you are taking including non-prescription medicines. Ask him what side effects you can expect. Also it would be wise to own a PDR. That is a book you can get or order in most book stores entitled, "Physicians Drug Reference". The PDR explains the side effects of each drug.

The *Pill Guide* is also available in bookstores, covers the most popular drugs and is only about $6.00.

If you experience any new and/or negative feelings while taking medication, call your doctor immediately. Your life might depend on it. And take only the recommended dosages.

Overdoses A Common Problem!

A federal report stated that over 80,000 people last year went to emergency rooms with prescription drug overdoses. Usually the drugs are tranquilizers, such as VALIUM, XANAX and sedatives.

Many doctors will prescribe a tranquilizer to any patient that asks. One doctor in New Mexico was responsible for 28% of ALL VALIUM prescribed to Medicare patients in the state.

Nine states have recognized the problem and have instituted a special three part prescription form. One copy is kept by the doctor, one goes to the pharmacy, and the other part goes to the state health agency. That way the states can track the doctors responsible for overprescribing like the one in New Mexico.

New System Cut Dangerous Drugs
By 50%!

As a result of this program in New York, California, Illinois and Texas, prescriptions for dangerous tranquilizers and sedatives dropped 35% to 50%. New York found that the reduction in just one class of sedative drug saved their Medicaid program $24 million the first year, according to a story in the *New York Times*.

Why don't all the other states have this prescription control system? Because of strong opposition from the fat cat drug company lobbyists who contribute heavily to the politicians.

The drug companies should be concerned. They stand to lose up to 50% of their sales of tranquilizers, sedatives and amphetamines which needlessly addict millions of people. We're talking about several BILLION dollars of lost sales.

80% Of Medical Procedures Don't Work!

The federal government has a department called the U.S. Office of Technology Assessment. They study and analyze the technological progress of various industries. According to their report on the medical field, almost 80% of conventional medical procedures don't work and have little scientific basis. Research shows that many people just heal despite what doctors do to them.

For example, three separate studies have shown that people don't live any longer after having bypass surgery. The heart surgeons don't like you having that knowledge. They gross $28 million A DAY doing bypass surgery, according to the *Wellness Letter*.

Per capita Americans have twice as many bypass surgeries as Canadians and five times as many as the people in France. Yet 20% more people in the United States die of heart disease than in Canada per capita..

More Competition Made Prices Go Up!

When anyone suggests that we do away with competition in the health services field, the drug companies and hospitals scream that prices will go up if there's no competition. What they know is that with no competition comes price controls.

The state of Arizona formerly controlled the number of hospitals that could do open heart surgery. During Reagan's "cut the regulations" campaign, the Arizona authorities got the idea that if more hospitals did open heart surgery, the price would drop.

Seven new hospitals in Phoenix joined the four existing facilities that offered open heart surgery. Within only one year the price rose over 50% and 35% MORE PEOPLE DIED!

84% Didn't Need Heart Surgery!

A Harvard study of heart patients found that 84% of those who were told by their doctors that they needed bypass surgery WERE FOUND NOT TO NEED IT!

The *Wellness Letter* reported that 17,500 patients die every year from this procedure. This clearly shows the awful greed of many doctors, and their complete disregard for human life! If the Harvard study is accurate, and we don't doubt it is; 84% or 14,875 people who were operated on last year could still be living—not dead!

The "science" of angioplasty, carotid endarterectomy and cancer chemotherapy is just "hope and a big medical bill." Cancer scientists admit that the success rate of chemotherapy is low for many types of cancer, but heart doctors are not so forthcoming about their hot new techniques.

Maybe This Is Why The Average Physician's Income Has Risen 44% In Just Eight Years!

Cardiac catherization is another popular procedure with which heart doctors pad their income. The cost is $4,000.00 to $5,000.00, but scientists say that very few are necessary out of the tens of thousands done each year.

Several uncomplicated and INEXPENSIVE stress tests will provide the same information about the patient. However, cardiac specialists love catherization, and so do the hospitals. Their share of the charge results in over 70% profit!

You Fill My Pocket, And I'll Fill Yours!

When a person is in a hospital, his or her doctor has the power to call in as many specialists as the doctor chooses. Often this goes way beyond the patient's needs.

A resident doctor at a major hospital says it is not unusual to see as many as five specialists on a case that is so simple NONE WERE NEED-ED.

The resident, Dr. Jones, (not his real name), said, "What they are doing is repaying favors. You fill my pocket, and I'll fill yours! And the insurance companies or Medicare have to pay for their 'consulting'."

Hospitals Drum Up Business For A New Department!

At the same hospital, a young intern fresh out of medical school told us that the administrator had billing clerks checking patients records to find the ones whose insurance would pay for "physical rehabilitation". The reason? The hospital had just opened a new physical rehabilitation ward! Who cares about patients needs? They are in this to make money!

Your Car Cost $1300 More Because Of Health Insurance Fees!

An analysis of Ford Motor Company's expenses reveals that the company spends about $1,300.00 PER CAR PRODUCED just to pay for health insurance. No wonder Japan can produce better cars for less money!

Every product you buy that is made in the United States is affected the same way Ford cars are. So you are paying to fatten the coffers of drug companies, hospitals and doctors; not only through the higher costs of products you buy, but also with the tax money that is spent on Medicare/Medicaid!

Padding Schemes Increase Insurance Company Costs Dramatically!

Our health system is so complicated because of doctors padding bills and doing unnecessary procedures that insurance companies require 10 TIMES THE NORMAL AMOUNT OF EMPLOYEES just to analyze claims.

For example, it takes as many claims administrators to authorize claims coming from doctors and hospitals at Blue Cross for 2.6 million policyholders as it does for THE ENTIRE CANADIAN HEALTH INSURANCE PROGRAM which covers over 26 million people!

Hospitals Are As Bad As Doctors!

It is no wonder that hospitals are as bad as doctors when it comes to padding insurance claims. Most hospitals are owned by a group of doctors, or they have a substantial interest therein.

The average 300 bed hospital in the United States has 36.4 billing employees. Yet in Canada, one billing clerk can handle the entire hospital!

Why the big difference? Several insurance company administrators told us that practically every claim from hospitals is loaded with inaccuracies and charges for unnecessary tests and procedures. Because of those problems, claims administrators must spend inordinate amounts of time on the phone with hospital billing clerks demanding explanations and documentation.

One way you can help is by demanding that someone go over every item on your bill and explain it to you when you check out of the hospital. Also try to keep track of every item that they deliver to your room or you—even Kleenex because you'll be charged (exorbitantly) for it.

The unfortunate part is that when you are sick and in a hospital (often doped up), you are neither in the mood nor the condition to pay attention to those details. It appears that that is obvious to hospital administrators, and they take advantage of the situation!

What Is The Answer?

Unfortunately our society has given doctors tremendous prestige and naive faith because we presume that they control life and death. That credibility has apparently carried over to the drug companies and hospitals. However, as we have shown, today the name of the game is money, and most doctors, drug companies and hospitals are out to get as much of it as they can.

They are totally out of control. The health costs in this country are a higher percentage of our gross national product than any other country in the world. The responsible parties are the doctors, drug companies and hospitals.

The Clintons are out to give every single person in this country health insurance which is a noble cause. Apparently they don't see that it will just make the doctors, drug companies and hospitals richer while the taxpayers foot the bill. We believe there are several ways to control these insidious profiteers and probably cut our health care costs by 75%!

Socialized medicine has certainly controlled and cut the costs dramatically in England and Canada. But the number employed by our government is already way too high. Socializing medicine would add tremendous numbers of government employees, and bureaucracies tend to grow rapidly.

There Is A Better System!

Almost a century ago, the leaders of this country began realizing that the utility companies (water, electricity) needed to be controlled because they had monopolies and could charge whatever they wanted. You can't get your electricity from another company because there isn't any.

Therefore they created laws that prevent utilities from raising their prices without first proving to government that their costs had increased. Also, the government regulated how much profit they could make which very low compared to drug companies.

Today, the company that sends gas into your home by pipeline is a utility (the oil companies aren't). Your local telephone (not long distance), some local bus companies and your cable TV company are all under the utility laws.

Doctors And Drug Companies Have A Monopoly!

The doctors and drug companies have a monopoly! They don't advertise their prices. Do you get on the phone and call doctors around town to see who has the best price? With the drug companies, you don't have a choice of what you pay for the prescriptions because the doctor dictates what you take. If that isn't a monopolistic situation, Webster better change the definition in his dictionary!

And they have abused their monopoly to the hilt. We are already paying much more than we can afford. Pity the poor person living on a few hundred dollars of Social Security payments each month. If they have the average four prescriptions, and have to pay 20% of their prescription costs under Medicare; they probably are doing without some other necessities such as good foods!

Here's Some Very Workable Answers To The Problem:

1. Put all drug companies under the utility laws controlling their price and profit.

2. Make it illegal to advertise a prescription drug to the public or distribute phony "public service" announcements and press releases, and enforce it with criminal penalties.

3. Restrict drug companies' advertising to doctors and hospitals to a package of test results on each drug once per year. In the case of generics, restrict them to a simple announcement of the availability of the substitute drug.

4. Make them eliminate their drug sales force which they call "detail persons".

5. Make it illegal to offer any inducement to doctors for prescribing drugs with criminal penalties.

6. Require them to cross test any drug against any other drug that possibly might be taken at the same time.

7. Make it mandatory that the potential side effects and dangers of other drugs taken at the same time be written in eighth grade English and Spanish, printed in 12 point type (the size of the text type in this book) and distributed with every prescription and refill.

8. Pay royalties to any government funded research center that creates a new drug that the drug company manufactures and sells.

The only realistic argument that we can envision by the drug companies is that the lack of advertising and sales people will eliminate competition. Well, the answer to that is that it most certainly will. But if a drug company patents a new drug, they have 17 years free of competition anyway.

And besides, we're discussing health, life and death. "Competition" doesn't seem very fitting for such sacred subjects.

Doctors Will Become Utilities, Too!

All states have utility commissions which audit and control the utilities' prices and profits. So it would be easy to put doctors under their control. The following are the changes we see that are necessary to control doctors:

1. Under the utility laws, control the net profit of a doctor relative to the number of patients handled and the amount of schooling they needed to reach their specialty.

2. Set a national standard price for all medical procedures, modifying it relative to regional cost differences. Allow it to increase only by the annual inflation figures.

3. Make it reasonably possible for doctors to attain an income in the upper 20% level. However, entrepreneurial doctors who employ other doctors or have more than one office should be rewarded for their extra effort and investment.

4. Make the three part prescription form mandatory in every state with monthly analyses of each doctor's prescription writing habits. Any doctors who overprescribe dangerous drugs will be prosecuted and their license revoked.

5. Require any doctors, who as a course of their business, prescribe drugs, tests or hospitalizations to sell their interests in any drug company, hospital, laboratory or any other profit center outside their normal practice. Make it illegal to have such interests.

6. Put all medical laboratories, hospitals, clinics and testing centers that deal with prescribing doctors under the utility laws.

7. Require all doctors who deal with patients to take a college course on nutrition before their license is renewed.

According to a recent study by the *American Journal of Nutrition*, the nation's doctors are not only ignorant about nutrition, but their arrogance thwarts the education of patients on the subject. Most doctors, when asked about vitamins or other nutrients, will say, "Just eat good foods. You don't need any vitamins or minerals."

The doctors apparently don't understand that today most vegetables, fruits and grains are grown in nutrient depleted soils by using chemical fertilizers. These chemical fertilizers don't replace many minerals needed by humans. Nor do they realize that food processing eliminates many vitamins.

8. Require doctors to complete a college course on preventive medicine, and demand that they discuss prevention measures with each patient. Perhaps have the federal health agencies create printed handouts for the majority of health disorders.

If we put our shoulders together and push our congresspeople to the wall, maybe we can solve this situation. We'll be sending a copy of this book to every congressional representative and senator shortly. However, the greatest impact will be your letters and calls to them.

Health Insurance Companies Becoming Aware Of The Value Of Preventive Medicine!

One of the nation's largest insurance companies has made a giant step forward in promoting preventive medicine. Mutual of Omaha announced that it would conduct a pilot program with people suffering from coronary artery disease who are candidates for bypass or other heart surgery.

The company will pay $3,500.00 per patient for a program developed by Dr. Dean Ornish, the director of Preventive Medicine Research Company of Sausalito, California. The program will be conducted at six locations around the country and last for two years.

Several hundred heart patients would eat a vegetarian diet low in fat and cholesterol, exercise moderately, be taught meditation techniques to relieve stress and attend support group meetings.

Terry Calek, senior vice president of public affairs at Mutual of Omaha, said, "What Cornish's program has done has proven that this is a viable alternative to costly bypass surgery and drug treatment."

Blue Shield and Blue Cross are also considering similar plans. Several HMOs began the trend by counseling patients on various reoccurring illnesses during the last year.

According to statistics, heart and blood vessel diseases kill more Americans than ALL OTHER DISEASES COMBINED! Dr. Cornish says, "I believe that 95% of those problems could be prevented or even reversed!"

Literally thousands of scientists and doctors throughout the world believe that Cornish's techniques apply to most illnesses and diseases that are not of genetic origin. Part of what you will learn in the following chapters will be about successful tests conducted under rigid scientific standards that prove you can prevent many illnesses.

You'll also learn, of course, about many other medicines for which you don't need a prescription. You should actively look for a doctor who understands the science of nutrition and preventive medicine. Consult with him or her before trying any of the suggestions in this book.

5

Smart Drugs, Memory Pills, And Natural Antidepressants Do Work!

Imagine the frustration, fear, and confusion associated with the realization that the sharp, active memory you once prided yourself on was, bit by bit, slipping away. Your first thought might be that the first stages of Alzheimer's Disease were setting in. With this possibility weighing heavily on your mind, it would be hard to keep a fog of depression from slipping slowly over you.

Perhaps you find lately that your usual ability to remember the phone numbers of dozens of friends and family is not what it used to be, or that your usual mental list of things to do, birthdays to remember and meetings to attend must now be written down constantly in your daily planner or on your calendar, or else you will forget. You do not feel that this situation is drastic enough to warrant worry about a debilitating disease, but you know that your usual sharp memory has been dulled slightly, and it bothers you.

One of these situations may have already happened to you. Each of us, as we age, finds that the sharp mind we took for granted can slowly, or much more quickly, ebb away. Sometimes it is as a result of a dreaded disease, such as Alzheimers'; sometimes simply the aging process that gradually dulls our mental acuity. If you are in this predicament, fear and dread follow quickly behind the first signs of a change, most probably because we are patterned to believe that memory loss, due to disease, aging, or of unknown origin is irreversible at present. Indeed, the depression that can follow from such a realization is easy to understand.

The Good News—Smart Drugs, Memory Pills And Natural Antidepressants Are Available!

There are drugs, nutritional supplements, vitamins, anti aging discoveries and natural antidepressants that are available. In some cases the substances can be obtained without a prescription. Many others are natural medicines and vitamins that have been around since humankind has existed. In still others there are drugs used regularly in foreign countries but held up by FDA red tape or the greed of doctors and drug companies looking for larger profits.

What follows is information about these drugs, natural substances, non-prescription medicines and vitamins that are available to you, as well as information regarding scientific testing done on these substances and how you can learn more about them.

Smart Drugs—Procaine, The Revitalizer!

In a recently published clinical study, Dr. Paul Luth of the Municipal Hospital Offenbach/Main, Germany, continues the examination of the drug Procaine (which was created in 1905) and its connection with brain metabolism.

Used for nearly fifty years as a local anesthetic because of its nontoxic properties and tissue compatibility, Procaine was originally investigated as a more encompassing drug by Dr. R. Leriche in the 1930's. When he began his studies of Procaine, he quickly realized that it could have a positive effect far beyond its initial use in surgery. Dr. Leriche reported that the injection of Procaine could be of great benefit to elderly people. Believing old age and its ensuing diseases to be caused by a nervous system which had been altered by harmful environmental causes, Dr. Leriche saw something in Procaine that could reverse that damage.

Geriatric Therapy—Dr. Leriche's Studies Are Continued!

Dr. Luth continued the studies of Dr. Leriche into the use of Procaine as a benefit to the elderly. In his studies, Luth administered Procaine by injection to a large test group of geriatric patients. These patients had diseases most common in the elderly, including hardening of the arteries (arteriosclerosis), arthritis, heart diseases, and diseases of the metabolism. After administering Procaine for an extended period of time, Dr. Luth was able to identify drastic changes in the appearance and behavior of these test patients.

Stage One Of Procaine Therapy— Skin Changes!

One of the first noticeable changes happened very quickly after Procaine therapy was begun and involved the appearance of the test patients' skin. The patient's skin very quickly appeared to sag less, and wrinkles and creases associated with old age were smoothed. Overall, the skin appeared tighter, giving the patients a more youthful, healthy appearance.

Irregular Heartbeats And High Blood Pressure Are Regulated And Sleep Is More Sound!

As Dr. Luth continued the Procaine therapy for his group, he found still more changes taking place; namely the regulation of heart arrhythmia and high blood pressure.

In the fourth stage of Procaine therapy, Dr. Luth's patients began to notice that their sleep was sounder, deeper and better. Many of these patients had complained of insomnia before beginning the study. Their overall feelings of well being and healthiness increased as their sleep patterns improved.

Stage Five—Psychological State Improves And Patients Feel Revived And Think More Clearly!

Dr. Luth found in stage five of Procaine therapy that his test patients showed a renewed interest in their surroundings, a marked improvement in memory, and that hearing problems and headaches that had plagued them regularly were eliminated.

Many of the patients, who had initially been diagnosed with hardening of the arteries (particularly in the brain) and Parkinson's Disease (a chronic, progressive nerve disease marked by tremors and weakness in resting muscles), showed a regression of their symptoms and disease related ailments.

Sixth And Final Stage Of Treatment— Effect On Blood Vessels And Degenerative Diseases!

In the final stage of Dr. Luth's Procaine treatment, Procaine was found to have a major effect on degenerative diseases about which his patients initially complained. Problems relating to hardening of the arteries, arthritis, and circulation in general lessened in patients who had previously had great difficulty in this respect.

What Makes Procaine Work Such Wonders?

Dr. Luth concludes his study by explaining the reason that Procaine therapy was so effective in his test patients and in test studies by other research scientists. The injection of Procaine stimulates the eventual production of dimethylaminoethanol, a salt that, when present in the body, produces return of memory, better sleep patterns, clearer thinking, and an overall feeling of well being and healthiness. In addition, dimethylaminoethanol reduces or eliminates symptoms of the brain most common in elderly people, including dizziness, headaches, and loss or change in hearing capacities.

Dr. Luth lastly concludes that the production of dimethylaminoethanol through Procaine therapy also shows extensive effects in non-geriatric patients. These younger patients show increased memory capacity, lessening of any type of continuous fatigue, and lessening or complete reduction of mild depression.

A Non-Prescription Substitute For Shots Of Procaine!

To create Procaine, chemists mix PABA and DMAE. Just a few years ago, a scientist named Dr. Hans Kugler wondered whether oral consumption of PABA and DMAE (which are common nutrients) would produce the same results as Procaine. In a double blind study at Roosevelt University in Chicago, Dr. Kugler proved his assumption was right. An American supplement manufacturer, Vita Industries, obtained the rights to his discovery. They added L-glutamine to the combination, and now market it as Gero Vita GH3, which does not require a prescription. You will learn more about the benefits of GH3 in the chapter on aging.

Another Smart Drug—Deprenyl!

Dr. Joseph Knoll, Chief of Pharmacology at Semmelwels Medical University, believes that, in Deprenyl, he has found a substance that reverses the devastation caused by such wasting diseases as Alzheimer's,

Parkinson's, and the everyday changes in memory retention and alertness that can come with aging. He is so sure of this "smart drug's" abilities to halt the aging process that he takes daily doses of it.

For some time Dr. Knoll's voice was the only one heard touting this wonder drug; but now, the voices of other scientists and physicians are joining his.

Studies On Rats Are Very Impressive!

Dr. Knoll's studies with male rats given Deprenyl reveal remarkable results. Rodents given the drug showed an increased ability to learn, and a renewed interest in sex into their old age; ages that were extended 210% longer than a control group that was given a placebo. If the same statistics were applied to humans, subjects receiving Deprenyl would have lived to be 150 years old!

Dr. Samuel Gershon, Vice President for Research in Health Sciences at the University of Pittsburgh, is one of the scientists who feel the tests in rats warrant a closer look at Deprenyl and its possible benefits for human subjects.

Positive Studies Move Deprenyl Closer To Becoming A Treatment For Human Age Related Diseases!

Findings similar to Dr. Knoll's have been repeated by researchers at the University of Toronto. These findings have added credence to Dr. Knoll's claims.

Six months after the Toronto results were published, the U.S. government approved the use of Deprenyl for the treatment of Parkinson's Disease. A human study done shortly after this governmental move showed that Deprenyl could actually retard the progression of Parkinson's.

Further Scientific Studies Show More Positive Results!

Dr. William Langston of the California Parkinson's Foundation in San Jose had long been searching for a drug such as Deprenyl. He reported in *Science Magazine* that patients in early stages of Parkinson's who were given Deprenyl took two times longer to develop more severe symptoms that required stronger drugs.

A large government study similar to Dr. Langston's showed identical results. Studies such as these provide even more powerful proof that using Deprenyl in early stage Parkinson's can slow the progression of its worst symptoms for extended periods of time.

How Does Deprenyl Work?

Dr. Knoll and his research fellows quickly discovered the reason that Deprenyl is able to have such strong effects on degenerative nerve diseases like Parkinson's Disease. They found that the drug blocks an enzyme called Monoamine Oxidase (MAO). This finding was significant, since MAO acts as an agent in the brain to staunch the production of excess dopamine, a chemical that transmits nerve impulses that heavily affect intricate muscle coordination, the immune system, physical energy, the ability to think, and short term memory. Dopamine levels drop in the average person at approximately 13% every ten years after the age of 45. By blocking MAO, Deprenyl allows more dopamine to be produced, and nerve impulses can flow more freely throughout the brain.

Since Parkinson's Disease destroys brain cells which produce dopamine, it was a logical decision to use Deprenyl to produce more dopamine to balance that loss.

Uses For Deprenyl Beyond Parkinson's Disease!

The next logical step is to apply Deprenyl to other diseases and conditions which result from a slowing of the flow of nerve impulses throughout the brain. Dr. Knoll feels that Deprenyl is a natural choice for use in safely treating depression, and might be applied as easily to Alzheimer's Disease and the ravages of premature senility.

Dr. Ira Shoulson, a neurologist at the University of Rochester, suggests that further clinical study is necessary. If those studies produce the same profoundly positive results, the next step should be to begin using Deprenyl to treat other degenerative brain diseases.

According to Dr. Stanley Fahn, a neurologist at Columbia-Presbyterian Medical Center in New York, tests being done on Parkinson's patients using a more potent but similar drug to Deprenyl which was developed by Hoffmann-LaRoches, Inc., could be the catalyst needed to move Deprenyl onward toward FDA approval, and Dr. Knoll's vision of its use in fighting other degenerative nervous diseases. If this drug, Hydergine, works as Deprenyl has, and slows down the progression of Parkinson's in its test patients; Dr. Fahn believes that a new class of medicine will be born.

One Of The First Drugs Tested To Combat Alzheimer's Disease Shows Promise!

Among the first drugs tested to combat Alzheimer's Disease, Hydergine was also one of the first to be given FDA approval as a treatment for deteriorating mental functions.

Despite the proven effects it has shown in increasing intelligence, learning ability, and short and long term memory, Hydergine is often rejected as a treatment for Alzheimer's, premature senility, and memory loss. Many American physicians do not use it in patient treatment. The reason behind this neglect may be that no one has been successful in proving how Hydergine works.

Regardless of this bit of missing information, according to Dr. Julian Whittaker, author of *Medical Memory Boosters and Brain Enhancers*, Hydergine does work. He states that it is not toxic, shows no serious side effects (barring some allergic reactions in a small portion of those treated), and is inexpensive. Hydergine is available via prescription from a physician, and all one needs to do is find a physician willing to prescribe it.

Alzene Vs. Other Alzheimer Treatments!

Dr. Shlomo Yehuda, an Israeli scientist educated at the Massachusetts Institute of Technology, developed the drug Alzene as a treatment for Alzheimer's Disease. In Alzene, Dr. Yehuda found a much less complex drug than the usual Alzheimer treatments, which have their foundations in the production of acetylcholine.

Acetylcholine is an intricate chemical which is responsible for the transmission of nerve impulses in the brain. Since Alzheimer's patients show very low levels of acetylcholine, their nerve impulse activity is also far lower. By supplying choline (from which acetylcholine is created), most drugs are meant to help the brain produce more acetylcholine, and thus increase nerve impulse activity.

The problem is in the amount of choline it takes to create enough acetylcholine to meet that task. Patients must take hundreds of pills per day, or, still worse, have small pumps implanted in their abdomens to send a supply of choline directly to the brain on a continual basis via a catheter.

Alzene—A Simple Drug With A Complex Task!

Alzene works in a more simple fashion than other drugs, with the same degree of success. It is a combination of two polyunsaturated fatty acids mixed with Vitamin E. The fatty acids, combined properly, can change the brain's nerve cell membrane and allow for a smoother flow of nerve impulses. In Alzene, Dr. Yehuda has discovered the correct combination of those fatty acids.

Results Of Testing Are Excellent And Drive Another Group Of Physicians Into Alzene Research!

Dr. Yehuda tested Alzene with 140 patients suffering from Alzheimer's. Of that group, nearly 70 showed better memory retention and clearer thinking ability after treatment with Alzene.

Those positive results came to the attention of Dr. Morton Shulman, who in 1987 founded Deprenyl Research in Toronto, Canada. Dr. Shulman began his research facility to study the very drug it is named after. His reasoning was, at least in part, very personal. Dr. Shulman suffers from Parkinson's Disease which by 1987 had taken its toll on him. He could not walk, talk, or drive a car because of the violent, uncontrolled tremors his body went through constantly.

Hearing that Deprenyl was being used throughout Europe to treat Parkinson's Disease successfully, Dr. Shulman obtained and took some of the drug himself. The following day, his tremors had lessened to the extent that he could walk again. He quickly secured the rights to market Deprenyl in Canada, and used an FDA loophole to make it available to patients in the U.S. as well.

Tests Of Alzene Begin In Canada!

Dr. Shulman is using the same artfulness to make Alzene immediately available to Canadians and to pave the way for its use in the United States. While Deprenyl Research runs tests on the drug in a double blind study, Dr. Shulman is using the compassionate use law available in Canada (which allows patients suffering from a disease to use an experimental drug while it is still being studied) to get Alzene into the hands of Alzheimer's patients.

Since 1988, the FDA has allowed the import of foreign drugs for private use which have not yet been approved in the U.S. All that Dr. Shulman needs to prove to satisfy the FDA is that Alzene works. Volunteer patients at Deprenyl Research are in the middle of the double blind study. Results are still forthcoming, but should they be as positive as Dr. Yehuda's, Alzene could join the ranks of what the world now calls "smart drugs".

DHEA Shows Promise In Battle Against Alzheimer's And Other Memory Disorders!

In studies published in 1990, another player entered the fight to treat Alzheimer's Disease and other memory disorders. Dr. Eugene Roberts, a research scientist in the Department of Neurobiochemistry at the Beckman Research Institute of the City of Hope in Duarte, California, reported in his paper, "Serum Steroid Levels of Those with Alzheimer's Disease," that DHEA showed tremendous effect in enhancing memory in young and old mice.

In his paper "Cognitive Effects of DHEA Replacement Therapy," Dr. Kenneth A. Bonnet, a research scientist in the Department of Psychiatry at New York University School of Medicine in New York City, reported similar findings. He injected young test mice with DHEA and found that they showed much higher levels of memory retention and recall. Upon injecting middle aged and old mice with DHEA, Dr. Bonnet found that their retention and recall skills, which had been remarkably lower than those of the young mice, increased to the same level as those of the young mice.

DHEA—Testing With A Human Subject Begins!

Dr. Bonnet reports of expanded studies in the paper mentioned above, detailing testing done with a 47 year old woman with lifelong multiple learning disabilities, low levels of memory retention, an inability to learn even the most simple information and reoccurring headaches. Among the diagnosis given to her prior to Dr. Bonnet's study were TMJ (temporal mandibular joint syndrome) and manic depression. Drugs used to treat this woman's problems before Dr. Bonnet's study were effective for short periods of time, but eventually her symptoms returned.

At the beginning of testing, the woman was given a standard five part intelligence test, and her sleep patterns were evaluated. The patient's recall abilities were reported as below normal, and an EEG showed evidence of poor sleep.

Low doses of DHEA were given to the patient for one week, then she was retested. The results showed an improvement in recall ability and the patient reported feeling better rested and sleeping more soundly. The woman also reported feeling an increase in clear thinking and ability to remember.

After one month, a higher dose of DHEA was given to the woman. Testing done after this increase showed more advanced ability to recall, with long term memory increasing also.

Results Of Testing Are Positive!

By the end of the testing period, the patient showed a marked increase in abilities. She was able to understand more clearly material presented to her an could apply that material, and could make judgments based on material presented to her.

Dr. Bonnet notes that the woman who was the subject of the test continued to take oral doses of DHEA and that a tolerance was not built up as was true of other drugs she took previously. In addition, for the first time in her 47 year life, after DHEA treatments began, the woman was able to begin and continue to run a small business.

The Possibilities For Using DHEA As A Treatment For Alzheimer's Disease Look Good!

In a study completed by Dr. C.R. Merril of the Laboratory of Biochemical Genetics at the National Institute of Mental Health in Bethesda, Maryland, 10 Alzheimer's patients were tested for blood serum levels of DHEA. These levels were compared to ten control subjects of the same age group who did not have Alzheimer's Disease. The results showed levels of DHEA in the Alzheimer's group to be 48% lower than the control group.

These findings are important because they reveal that Alzheimer patients have much less DHEA than those without the disease. The 47 year old test patient from Dr. Bonnet's study also showed extremely low levels of DHEA when testing began. It is entirely possible that Alzheimer patients may be able to benefit from DHEA treatment as did the female test patient. Studies into this possibility are now underway.

Natural Substance Shows Promise In Fighting The Deterioration Of Alzheimer's!

Italian researchers, led by Dr. Alberto Spagnoli of the Mario Negri Institute in Milan, have begun a year-long double blind study of a natural compound called acetyl-L-carnitine which has been reported to slow the deteriorating mentality common to Alzheimer patients. Of the 130 patients involved in the study, the 63 who received acetyl-L-carnitine have shown improved attention span, better long term memory, and increased verbal ability with no side effects. The 67 patients involved in the same study who received placebos showed no improvement.

Acetyl-L-carnitine works as a nerve cell stimulator, increasing the cell's ability to produce acetylcholine, proteins and new cell membranes.

Tests done on animals have proven all of Dr. Spagnoli's claims, showing that acetyl-L-carnitine stimulated nerve cells to produce proteins, new cell membranes and acetylcholine.

Tests To Be Done Prior To Seeking FDA Approval!

Dr. Susan Sauer of Sigma-Tau Pharmaceuticals, Inc. in Gaithersburg, Maryland, has gathered 400 Alzheimer's patients for a similar one year study to be carried out at 27 Alzheimer research centers throughout the country. Upon completion of the study, Sigma-Tau plans to seek FDA approval to sell the drug in the U.S.

An Amino Acid Begins The Test Process!

The amino acid, EDTA (ethylenediaminetetraaceticacid), is also currently being tested with Alzheimer's patients in the United States Since studies began, EDTA has shown positive results in increasing comprehension and memory in the test groups.

PAC—An Antioxidant To Protect Brain Cells!

Another substance showing promise is proanthocyanidine (PAC). It is a dietary antioxidant that crosses the blood brain barrier to protect the brain against free radicals.

Researchers feel that PAC can also aid in strengthening capillaries, thereby regulating blood pressure. Rats bred to be prone to high blood pressure and strokes lived considerably longer when given PAC. In addition, other test animals that were given chemicals to scar and damage their blood vessels showed no sign of damage if given PAC beforehand.

Dr. Peter Rohdewald of the Pharmacology Institute of the University of Munster in Germany states that PAC is not toxic, and has been used in Indian cultures for centuries with no reports of toxicity.

L-Glutamine—Brain Fuel!

In a paper entitled *"Fourteen Doctors Confirm L-Glutamine Improves I.Q.,"* Dr. Richard Passwater explains that the brain actually needs two types of "fuel". Until recently, doctors knew of only one type, glucose; but recent studies have proven that another compound exists and also nourishes the brain. That compound is L-glutamine.

L-glutamine affects brain cell activity. When the brain is not supplied sufficiently with this compound, minor brain damage can occur.

Doctors Rave About L-Glutamine's Uses!

L-glutamine appears to be beneficial in many different ways. In his book, *Mega Nutrients for Your Nerves*, Dr. H.L. Newbold states that L-glutamine can be used to relieve depression, impotence, and works as an all around energizer.

Dr. L.L. Rogers, in *Texas Reports on Biology and Medicine*, found that L-glutamine improved I.Q. scores of mentally retarded children.

A Nutrient That Is More Effective Than Choline!

As we mentioned earlier, acetylcholine is a complex chemical which acts as a neurotransmitter in the brain. Acetylcholine is a product of choline, therefore many drugs used to reverse degenerative brain diseases include choline. The problem is in the amount of choline needed to create quantities of acetylcholine that will be effective. Huge amounts of this substance must be ingested or directly injected in order for positive results to be seen.

There is, however, another nutrient which is more easily passed across the blood-brain barrier than choline and appears to be just as effective. It is dimethylaminoethanol (DMAE). Dr. R. Hochschild, in his article *"Effect of DMAE On The Life Span Of Senile Male A/J Mice,"* reports that

DMAE is far superior to choline in its ability to reach the location within cells where production of membranes occurs.

Although DMAE is found in such foods as anchovies and sardines, one would have to consume large quantities of these foods in order to see substantial benefit. An easier method is to take dietary supplements.

Dr. H. Murphree states in his article *"The Stimulant Effect of DMAE in Human Volunteer Subjects,"* that DMAE produced clearer mental concentration, increased muscle tone, and positive changes in sleep patterns in the patients he studied.

Dr. Ross Pelton, author of *Mind Food and Smart Pills*, found that his subjects showed better moods, improved memory and learning ability, and higher intelligence after treatment with DMAE.

The Oldest Living Tree On Earth Holds Promise As An Extraordinary Medicine!

The ginkgo biloba or maidenhair tree, as it is sometimes known, is the oldest living tree on Earth. Originally only found in China, ginkgo biloba has been on this planet since before the Ice Age. Fossilized leaves of the tree have been carbon dated to as far back as 250,000,000 years. It is completely unaffected by the withering effects of blight and air pollution. A ginkgo sprouted less than 100 feet from ground zero in the spring after the dropping of the atomic bomb at Hiroshima.

Ginkgo biloba trees have been imported all over the globe. They can be found in Europe, South America, and in cities all over the United States. Some trees living today have been reported to be over 1,000 years old.

It is not surprising that people have used an extract from this remarkable tree's leaves as a medicine for over 5,000 years. The extract is used in clinics and hospitals all over Europe and Asia, making it possibly the most widely prescribed medicine there. Sales of the extract total $500 million per year in Europe alone. The prescription sales in France make up 1.5%

of prescriptions written per year. In 1989, 10 million prescriptions were written for ginkgo throughout the world.

Natural Nutrient Extracted From Ginkgo Biloba Has Antiaging Properties!

Ginkgo biloba extract has been shown in global testing to be an effective antiaging medicine. It works by widening blood vessels to the brain, heart, and extremities, and acts as a protectant against free radicals, which can cause tissue damage. In March 1988, *The New York Times* reported that laboratory synthesis of ginkgo biloba could, in time, lead to its use to fight Alzheimer's disease and numerous circulatory problems.

Chinese medical records which go back to the year 2,800 B.C., show ginkgo biloba's use in treatment of many age related complaints, including circulation problems, memory loss and mental deterioration.

Physician's Feel Ginkgo Biloba May Be Effective In Fighting Alzheimer's And Other Age-Related Diseases!

Dr. C.H. Warden reported in *The Journal of Biological Chemistry* that ginkgo biloba, in the proper dosages, may have a strong effect on preventing hardening of the arteries.

Reports from Dr. J.L. Wood show that ginkgo biloba can be effective in reducing the symptoms of illnesses like Alzheimer's.

Dr. Ross Pelton states that tests done on healthy subjects showed improved memory retention after doses of ginkgo biloba were given. Tests given in short term memory retention and memory of abstract words before and after treatment with ginkgo biloba showed increased abilities in both these areas after treatment was completed.

In a long term, six month test with older Alzheimer patients, Dr. A. Little reported that patients showed improved memory and retention after being treated with ginkgo biloba.

By Taking Vitamins We Can Increase Memory Capacity!

For memory enhancement and mental functions, Dr. Julian Whitaker, author of *Medical Memory Boosters and Brain Enhancers*, recommends a diet rich in B-complex vitamins, vitamins C and E, and lecithin/choline, for improved memory enhancement and mental functions.

These vitamins are available in such foods as citrus fruits (C), whole grains (B-complex), and green leafy vegetables (E); but most individuals do not regulate their diets well enough to get the proper amounts of these vitamins through diet alone. In order to best ensure that we are receiving the proper amounts of these important vitamins, Dr. Whitaker recommends that vitamin supplements in capsule form be taken daily.

Mental Function Can Be Affected By Vitamin Intake!

According to Dr. Whitaker, these vitamins effect our mental functions in the following ways:

B (thiamine): Protects nerve tissue against the harmful effects of alcohol, tobacco, and, most important, the aging process itself.

B_3 (niacin): Acts to improve memory. A study involving B_3 showed patients in all age groups given 141 mg of the vitamin daily reported increased memory function. It should be noted that B_3 is very high in acid and should be taken on a full stomach to avoid stomach problems.

B_5 (pantothenic acid): It is a powerful antioxidant, is important during high stress periods, and acts as a stamina enhancer. It should be noted that Dr. Whitaker reports that too large a dose can cause diarrhea. Should this occur, reducing the intake of B_5 will probably take care of the problem, and levels can then be increased by small increments.

B_6 (pyridoxine): Helps to produce nerve transmitters and enhance mental functions.

B_{12} (cyanocobalamin): Aids in learning abilities; in particular, absorbing new material.

Connections Between B Complex Vitamin Deficiency And Mental Disfunction And Illness!

According to Dr. William J. Evans, Chief of the Human Physiology Laboratory at the USDA Human Nutrition Research Center on Aging, and author of the book *Biomarkers*, results from a study financed by the USDA show that concentration levels of B_6, B_{12}, and folic acid drop as people age. Lower levels of these vitamins can cause decreases in patient alertness and memory capacity.

When Dr. Evans' subjects were given vitamin supplements to bring the levels up to normal, they showed increased alertness and better memory. As a result of his findings, Dr. Evans recommends an increase in the Recommended Daily Allowance of B_6, B_{12}, and folic acid in elderly patients.

Studies completed by Dr. Whitaker have also determined that deficiencies in B_{12} can lead to mental illness. A study done on mentally retarded children showed that after being given large does of B-complex vitamins, I.Q. levels increased by 10.2%.

Vitamin C Helps In Production Of Nerve Transmitters And Cell Structures!

Vitamin C has been proven to aid in producing nerve transmitters and building cell structures. A study of school children from kindergarten age to college level found that by increasing vitamin C levels in blood plasma by 50% , I.Q. levels also increased by 3.6%. The same study applied to retarded children showed increased I.Q. levels of 20 points or greater.

Vitamin E And Lecithin/Choline Affect Brain Cells In A Positive Way!

According to Dr. Whitaker, Vitamin E blocks the oxidation of cell molecules. It is believed to help slow down the aging process.

Lecithin/choline is the building block from which every cell membrane in the human body is made. It is essential in the process of nerve transmission and in producing neurotransmitters. Cells in the nerves and brain require high volumes of it in order to grow and survive.

Tests done by Dr. Hardo Sorjatz of the Institute for Physiology in Dormstad, Germany, showed patients taking eight grams of lecithin/choline per day scored higher on both written and oral memory tests, compared to patients taking a placebo.

It should be noted that, according to Dr. Whitaker, lecithin/choline should always be taken with vitamin B$_5$ (pantothenic acid).

Depression—Prozac And Its Link To Violent Behavior And Suicidal Tendencies!

As we stated at the beginning of this chapter, the toll taken on memory capacity and mental acuity by the aging process and diseases like

Alzheimer's can often result in severe mental depression. When patients notice changes in mental capacity, the fear that results can quickly turn into feelings of hopelessness.

Until recently, for cases of severe depression the medical world has prescribed what was believed to be a miracle drug. That drug is called Prozac. Reports of violent behavior and severe suicidal impulses began to surface in connection with patients taking Prozac in 1990. Until this time, Prozac was considered a wonder drug and had become the nation's best-selling antidepressant, according to a report in the *New York Times*.

In the same *New York Times* article, the nonprofit Public Citizen Health Research Group was reported to have petitioned the FDA to strongly caution the medical world regarding evidence that Prozac could cause impulsively violent and suicidal thoughts and actions in some patients taking the drug. The group even asked the FDA to require warning labels on Prozac, warning patients of possible of violent side effects.

Statistics Of Violent And Suicidal Acts Linked To Prozac Are Incredibly Disturbing!

In 1990, Dr. Martin Teicher, a research psychiatrist at Harvard University, reported on six patients who showed intense and during Prozac therapy.

As of June, 1992, the Citizen's Commission of Human Rights reported Prozac as having the largest number of adverse drug reactions of any drug in history (23,067, which included 1,436 suicide attempts and 1,313 deaths). These figures are particularly telling when compared to the nation's average of adverse drug reactions to antidepressant prescription drugs, which is 1,744.

The Reason Behind The Medical World's Continued Use Of Prozac!

With statistics such as those listed above, it would seem amazing that the medical world would even consider the continued prescription of Prozac as treatment for depression. It becomes less amazing when one looks at the profit the drug's producer, Eli Lilly & Company has made on the sale of Prozac. In 1990 alone, Lilly showed a profit of $385 million on the sale of Prozac.

With such huge profits involved, it is easy to see how strongly one of the nation's largest pharmaceutical giants might push the continued use of a drug like Prozac to U.S. physicians.

With the possible dangers of Prozac clearly evident, the question becomes, "What other alternatives exist to fight depression?" The answer is that there are many safe and natural antidepressants available.

Tyrosine—A Natural Antidepressant Amino Acid!

Dr. Earl Mindell, stated that the amino acid tyrosine showed amazing results in tests on patients with severe mental and emotional depression. According to Dr. Mindell, tyrosine acts against depression by releasing catecholamine, an organic compound that stimulates nerve cells in the brain to produce epinephrine and norepinephrine. Both of these substances show positive results in acting against emotional depression by creating a non-narcotic sensation of calmness in patients.

Another substance released in treatment with tyrosine is dopamine, which we talked about earlier in this chapter. Dopamine transmits nerve impulses throughout the brain and is also believed to produce a calming effect in depressed patients.

Studies done on tyrosine by Dr. Alan J. Gelenberg of Harvard Medical School as reported in the *American Journal of Psychiatry* also show the tranquilizing effects that tyrosine can have on patients suffering from depression. Dr. Gelenberg reported that patients showed positive responses when given oral doses of tyrosine. Three out of five patients in another study conducted by Dr. Gelenberg showed reductions in depression by at least 50% after receiving oral doses of tyrosine for a period of four weeks. Control patients in the same study who received a placebo showed such reductions in only one of four cases.

DLPA (Phenylalanine)—Another Amino Acid Which Can Be Used To Treat Depression!

DLPA is another amino acid which has shown promise in fighting clinical depression. DLPA produces nerve transmitters, which regulate a person's sense of well-being and help in mood elevation.

Melatonin—A Substance That Can Fight Depression In The Elderly!

One type of depression that is particularly common in the elderly is called SAD (Seasonal Affective Disorder). Patients suffering from SAD become depressed during times of the year when daylight hours are diminished. Therapy using high-intensity light has been proven to relieve these feelings of depression. This light therapy has also been proven to increase the levels of the substance melatonin in SAD patients tested during darkened cycles.

Melatonin can be taken as a supplement to counter depression. It is available without prescription at minimal expense and has shown no evidence of toxicity in patients tested.

Biotin—Tests Show Its Effectiveness As An Antidepressant!

As long ago as 1940, biotin, a component of the vitamin B complex, has been the subject of experiments with clinical depression. In a report in

The Journal of the American Medical Association, Dr. V.P. Sydenstricker reported on an experimental study which he performed on four healthy patients. The subjects were given a diet rich in all nutrients except biotin. After living on this diet for 10 weeks, all the subjects showed severe signs of depression and exhaustion, as well as nausea, anorexia and complaints of muscle pain. Immediately after supplements of biotin were given to these subjects, all symptoms vanished.

Dr. R. Levenson reported a study he did in 1983 of a patient who was experiencing depression, as well as nausea, insomnia, headaches, and an overall feeling of fatigue. After five days of treatment with supplements of biotin, the patient showed a lessening of these symptoms, and continued treatment with biotin completely eliminated his feelings of depression.

One Of Europe's Answers To Prozac— Hypericum Extract!

Although there appears to be a trend in the U.S. toward the use of more natural medications by physicians, European physicians still seem to be more receptive to treatments using nature's own drugs.

One such medication, hypericum extract, is used successfully in European countries as a natural antidepressant. Six woman from the ages of 55 to 65, suffering from depression, were treated with the extract in a German study. The six patients were tested before and after treatment to evaluate depression and anxiety levels, and were found to show highly decreased levels of depression and anxiety after the treatment was completed.

Their blood levels also showed a greater quantity of dopamine after treatment. Dopamine levels are known to increase in successful antidepressant therapy.

Natural And Alternative Therapies To Prevent Brain Deterioration And Depression Do Exist And Can Be An Option!

There are a multitude of treatments and medications available through prescription and over the counter to treat brain deterioration and depression. What we have hoped to show is that changes in thought amongst worldwide medical personnel, as well as new discoveries and treatments, are opening up entirely new options for the treatment of age related diseases and conditions related to brain deterioration, as well as the depression which so often accompanies it.

Health care is changing every day, and we believe the information contained in this chapter is a good example of how such change can be extremely beneficial for you; and open up new options in treatment.

Sources of Substances Mentioned In This Chapter:

The following are available from health food and vitamin stores:
  Acetyl-L-carnitine (ask for carnitine).
  DLPA (phenylalanine)
  DMAE (dimethyl-amino-ethenol) also an ingredient in GeroVita GH3.
  Ginkgo biloba
  L-Glutamine
  PAC (proanthocyanidine) It may be called phycotene.
  Tyrosine

Vitamins:
  B_1 (thiamin)
  B_3 (niacin)
  B_5 (pantothenic acid)
  B_6 (Pyridoxine)
  B_{12} (cyanocobalamin)
  C (ascorbic acid)

E
Lecithin
Choline

Mail order sources:

Melatonin -
 Available only from Life Extension Foundation of Hollywood,
 Florida - 1-800-841-5433 or 305-966-4886.

DHEA (dehydroepiandrosterone)
 May be available from Belmar Pharmacy, 8015 W. Almeda Ave.
 Suite 100, Lakewood, CO 80226, 1-800-525-9473; and
 College Pharmacy, 833 N. Tejon St.,
 Colorado Springs, CO 80903, 1-800-748-2263

 Vita Potencia, made by Gero Vita International, contains naturally-
occuring DHEA from Mexican wild yam.

Nutrients listed under health food and vitamin stores may also be pur-
chased by mail from the following:
 Indiana Botanic Gardens
 P.O. Box 5, Dept.
 Hammond, IN 46325,
 219-947-4040

The following is for experimental use and only available to scientists:
 EDTA (ethylenediaminetetra-acetic acid)

Drugs:
 Alzene: By prescription
 Deprenyl: By prescription only
 Procaine: By prescription only.
 Procaine substitute (no prescription needed) Gero Vita GH3:
 Available from Gero Vita International,
 Dept. Z101, 2255-B Queen Street East #820,
 Toronto, Ontario M4E 1G3, Canada,
 or call (800) 825-8482.

Miscellaneous Health Problems

Stop Strokes, Leg Cramps, Gum Disease—But Not Colds!

Scientific research has discovered that vitamins A and C, taken together with a natural substance called rutin, cut the likelihood of strokes!

Rutin comes from citrus fruit. It's an example of what are known as bioflavonoids, which are found in citrus pith. In other words, rutin is all natural and completely safe.

It is surprisingly effective. Your odds of suffering a stroke when you combine rutin with vitamins A and C are cut by a whopping 75%!

This was the conclusion of research done at Cornell University. A separate study done at Washington University confirmed the finding.

Simple Solutions For Leg Cramps!

Medical researchers know that calcium lowers blood pressure, improves circulation, and helps relax muscles. In fact, contracted muscle fibers can't extend without it. So perhaps it should come as no surprise that calcium supplements have been demonstrated to ease even the most stubborn leg cramps!

But it has to be the right kind of calcium supplement. Researchers advise trying different brands until you find the one that works best for you.

Phosphorous Can Help!

It might also help to take a phosphorous supplement with your calcium, research reveals. Two good examples of phosphorous supplements are Nutri-Dyne's Orthophos and Standard Processes Phosfood. Either one helps balance calcium and phosphorous levels, so that the right amount of calcium gets to muscles, scientists say. Both phosphorous and calcium are natural and sold over-the-counter.

An Even Faster Solution!

If all this fails, or if it's an emergency and you need a quicker fix, Dr. Donald Cooper told the journal *Cortlandt Forum* that pinching your top lip between thumb and index finger for 20 to 30 seconds will alleviate a cramp 9 out of 10 times. "Sometimes it may take longer," said Dr. Cooper. But, he advised, "don't knock it until you've tried it."

Another, longer-term solution is to improve blood circulation so that the calcium in your system can be used properly:

- Step 1: Exercise, which enlarges blood vessels in your muscles.
- Step 2: Take vitamin B_5, also called niacin. Studies show that a gram of niacinamide, a form of the vitamin, taken daily, helps open blood vessels.
- Step 3: If you smoke, quit. Smoking contracts blood vessels.

Help For Ailing Teeth And Gums!

Mouthwash isn't just for kissing anymore. Recent research proves that certain kinds of mouthwash, used correctly, reduce plaque—and therefore, tartar, tooth decay, gum disease and, in all likelihood, your dental bills!

We spend about $7.5 billion on dental visits every year in this country, most of which is for these kinds of preventable ailments.

Plaque!

What *is* plaque? Lick your teeth. Feel coated or sticky? That's plaque. It's invisible and comes primarily at night from normal bacteria, saliva, and food particles. Left untreated, it will harden and become tartar. And plaque plus tartar leads to any number of more serious diseases—gingivitis, for example, which is swollen, infected gums; or periodontitis, a gradual erosion of dental bone and tissue culminating in possible tooth loss!

Mouthwash May Save Teeth!

Brushing and flossing, of course, remain important to oral hygiene, but often they are not enough. Many plaque-reducing mouthwashes are readily available in any supermarket, while others from overseas have only recently come to these shores. They may be harder to find, but are worth the search!

Here are the key active ingredients to look for: Propolis, widely tested and used in the former Soviet Union, is a sticky substance bees make from tree sap and use to line honeycombs. This "bee glue" has been shown in German studies not only to reduce plaque and gingivitis, but to heal gum injuries, tooth extractions and gangrene of the mouth.

In Germany, China, and Poland, propolis can be found in many mouthwashes and toothpastes. In this country, you may have to look in specialty stores and catalogues (see end of chapter). Propolis and its extracts come in powders, creams or pills, so it can be applied externally, gargled or swallowed.

CoEnzyme Q, Or CoQ!

This is a natural substance found in healthy gum tissue but not in diseased gums. Daily CoQ treatments have been shown to produce innumerable benefits. Dr. Edward Wilkinson said in *Biomedical and Clinical Aspects of Coenzyme Q* that 50 mg to 70 mg a day reduced pain, inflammation, and bleeding in his patients' gums; sometimes, it even eliminated the need for oral surgery!

Sanguinarine, The Nigerian Chewing Stick!

Another natural product derived from plants, sanguinarine has been used widely in Nigeria and is now available here in common mouthwash. It not only reduces plaque but makes more visible whatever plaque remains. So while using it may dull your pearly whites, it will also make problem areas easier to spot and clean.

Cetylpyridinium Chloride Goes For The Source!

A big name for a powerful plaque fighter, this one works by combating plaque-causing bacteria. When combined with domiphen bromide, results last even longer.

Volatile Oils Work Wonders!

Finally, volatile oils such as eucalyptol and menthol are proven to work well against not only plaque but also gingivitis.

The Common Cold: Children Beware!

Americans spent $1.4 billion on over-the-counter cold medicines in 1991, with over 66% of households reporting they stock four to eight different types in their home medicine cabinets. With more than 800 brands to choose from, it is a very big business indeed!

But a new study indicates there is more than a little truth in the old saying, "A cold will go away in a week if you treat it, but will take seven days if you don't."

Cold Research Called "Shoddy!"

Dr. Michael B.H. Smith, of Izaak Walton Killam Children's Hospital in Halifax, Canada, reviewed all the scientific research on these cold medications done since 1950 and found, "There's a lot of shoddy research in this area."

Of 106 studies, only 27 were scientifically valid. From those, Smith concluded that while cold medicines can relieve symptoms for adolescents and adults, they do nothing for children—especially children under six, who tend to get the most colds.

Findings for children aged 6 to 13 were "weak," he said, because they neglected to take into account the placebo effect, which is considered strong, particularly in youths, according to a Johns Hopkins University study.

Cold Medicines May Be Dangerous For The Youngest!

And as for children under six, "the potential for side effects," Smith reported, are such that "there is no reason to have these products available" for them.

What's more, the American Association of Poison Control Centers says over 73,000 kids under six overdosed on cold medicines in 1990—the number two cause of childhood overdose, after analgesics!

Cause For Hope!

But there is hope. Scientifically valid studies in Poland, Bulgaria, Romania, and Russia, which did take into account the placebo effect, found that propolis—the same all-natural "bee glue" that's good for your teeth and gums—has an amazing impact on the common cold even in the youngest children!

Whether diluted in water and gargled, then swallowed; taken as a nasal spray; or mixed with honey (or anything sweet) for children—propolis has been proven to work so fast on a variety of infections it may well put the standard antihistamine and decongestant business out of business!

Relief From Kidney Stones!

You can drink six to eight glasses of water a day and still get kidney stones. If they remain unpassed, your doctor will probably recommend something called lithotripsy treatment—a process of blasting the stones with sound waves until they shatter, using a machine that costs some $3 million. In many cases, doctors also prescribe surgery. Your bill: tens of thousands of dollars.

Beat The High Cost Of Kidney Stone Treatment!

Dr. William Boyce, a Virginia-based physician, says "the promoters of lithotripsy" have been calling the shots too long. He maintains there are proven alternatives. And he is not alone.

In Los Angeles, University of Southern California urology professor and director of the Kidney Stone Department at Burbank's St. Joseph's Medical Center, Dr. Peter D. Fugelso points out, "92 percent of kidney stones are made of calcium or calcium products. And almost all of the calcium in your diet comes from dairy products." So cutting down on how much cheese you eat, for example, might be a good idea.

Another, he says, is to check your antacid remedy. Some of them even boast of how much calcium they offer!

He also maintains that it's not how much water you drink a day that counts. "It's the amount of urine [you make]," he says. Drink "enough [water] to pass 2 quarts of urine a day."

No Chocolate—Or Spinach!

Dr. Brian L.G. Morgan, at Columbia University College of Physicians and Surgeons' Institute of Human Nutrition, points out that 60 percent of all kidney stones are made up of calcium combined with oxalates—a substance found in certain types of produce—which normally passes through your system with no problem. He recommends restricting your intake of oxalate-rich foods. These include beans, beets, green peppers, spinach, and, yes, cocoa.

Magnesium Can Help!

At the Harvard Medical School, Dr. Edwin Prien and Dr. Stanley Gershoff go further. Following up on experiments done in Sweden, they confirmed that magnesium can help dissolve these calcium-oxalate stones. Magnesium apparently bonds with oxalates as well as calcium does, but the magnesium-oxalate combination does not make stones!

What's more, the Harvard researchers found back in 1974 that vitamin B_6 slows oxalate formation in the first place. So, taken together in even moderate doses of 300 mg and 10 mg respectively, magnesium oxide and vitamin B_6 "are effective in prevention of recurrence of idiopathic calcium-oxalate stones," they concluded. Indeed, their studies showed incidence of these stones fell a whopping 92 percent!

Eat Right!

Eating a low-fat, high-fiber diet is a good plan for preventing kidney stones, too. Research shows it provides a healthy dose of magnesium and vitamin B_6. Also, vitamin C, which had been thought to contribute to kidney stones, has been found to help prevent them! It raises the acid level in your urine, which assists in dissolving stones.

An Alternative To
Dying Of Emphysema!

Emphysema is a killer. A disease of the lungs, it is especially common among smokers. Others get it too, though, in our air-polluted society. Doctors may be able to prolong the life of emphysema sufferers, but generally they're just delaying the inevitable.

The Dallas-based International Bio-Oxidative Medical Foundation offers a new treatment for emphysema and other bronchial conditions—a treatment reportedly proven to work better than the oxygen, cortisone, and drug therapies doctors traditionally rely on, in vain. Perhaps best of all, it's comparatively simple and inexpensive.

A Two-Step Process For
Breathing Easier!

The first step of the bio-oxidative treatment involves intravenous doses of hydrogen peroxide. How does it work? Dr. Charles Farr likens the effect to what happens with Alka-Seltzer: Fluid in your lungs becomes effervescent as oxygen moves the bronchial mucus. At first, you cough and cough, he reports. But the fluids are loosened, and soon the lungs feel clearer, producing a kind of catharsis that is said to be a great relief in many patients!

A Cure From The Past,
Rediscovered!

The second step is photoluminescence of the blood, which means shining ultraviolet light on a sample of your blood. Sound hokey? Before the discovery of penicillin, it was a chief subject of medical research for a variety of ailments!

The combined bio-oxidative treatment is reported to work particularly well in folks who have bronchiectasis, a disease characterized by pockets of pus in the lungs. Unlike emphysema, bronchiectasis is not generally fatal. Symptoms, however, are similar for both. Sufferers are weak, cough incessantly and hopelessly and tend to be thin and pallid—often vaguely blue-skinned. Secondary infections, such as pneumonia, are common.

No More Infections!

Infections are made even more likely by the cortisone treatments doctors conventionally prescribe. Cortisone inhibits the body's natural immune system.

Asthmatics are especially probable candidates for emphysema. So is anyone who has been exposed to unusual amounts of factory smoke, coal dust, or other pollutants.

No Smoking, Please!

Quitting smoking remains the single best way to prevent emphysema, bronchiectasis or any other lung disease. Not only is smoking itself harmful, but reports indicate it renders you extra vulnerable to environmental pollutants.

Bio-Oxidative therapy, then, is a much-needed treatment, providing hope for the many who are literally drowning in their own pus and mucus. Perhaps they will finally be able to breathe a sigh of relief.

Yeast Infections!

Yeast infections affect men as well as women, the culprit being a naturally occurring bacteria called *Candida albicans*. You'll know you've got it if your mouth or skin bleeds easily, peels, or excretes a white goo— though, of course, the most common form is vaginitis.

What causes yeast infections? Antibiotics can, since they upset the balance of bacteria in your body. So can an imbalance in your nutritional intake, according to some.

Dr. Laurence Urdang says doctors generally prescribe costly anti-fungal drugs as a solution. But evidence is mounting that there is a better way.

Alternatives To
Antifungal Medication!

In Monterey, Mexico, 20 women with vaginal yeast infections douched with a natural grapefruit-seed extract twice daily for three days, and found it did the trick. According to Dr. Luis E. Todd, 15 of them felt better after the first treatment!

A study in Germany with 25 women confirmed the finding, Dr. G. Ionescu reports.

In Brazil, writes Dr. Michael Tierra, physicians recommend a tea made from the bark of a tree called the *pau d'arco*.

And in this country, Dr. John Parks Trowbridge explains that a form of vitamin B, called biotin, can boost the body's ability to fight off and recover from a variety of diseases, not the least of which are yeast infections! "Biotin can help prevent the conversion of the yeast form of Candida to its fungal form," he writes in *The Yeast Syndrome*.

Studies Confirm: Certain Foods Help!

He also tells of a University of Massachusetts study that concluded that simple garlic—whole clove or the extract—is a good weapon against yeast infections.

And in his *"Therapeutic Properties of Acidophilus Milk,"* Dr. C.D. Khedkar explains the benefits of this natural, yogurt-like drink for fighting off "several human pathogens."

Trowbridge concurs. Acidophilus creates various enzymes, he writes, "all of which retard the growth of *Candida albicans*. [They work like] bulwarks in the anti-yeast holistic therapy program."

Nature's Solutions
In A Convenient Package!

What does all this mean? Nature provides many simple, safe solutions for yeast infections! And unlike drugs, these remedies offer virtually no possibility of side effects.

A homeopathic treatment, called Candida Guard, contains all the above natural remedies, plus more.

Candida albicans is a natural and usually beneficial yeast that lives in all of us. When it becomes an irritant, scientists have found it means something has disrupted the delicate natural arrangement of your system.

A Safe Way To Return
To A Healthy State!

What better way to deal with these disruptions, than a natural solution that will enable your body to restore its own equilibrium?

Dr. Trowbridge says, "A victim of the yeast syndrome must return to a symbiotic balance with friendly bacteria in order to discourage the invasion of excess *Candida albicans* parasites."

Nonprescription Remedies
Save Money!

William Soller, of the Nonprescription Drug Manufacturers Association, suggests "A number of analyses have shown that O.T.C.'s [over-the-counter drugs] not only provide effective and safe relief from a large number of common, everyday maladies...but also provide a defined and significant cost savings."

His 1991 figures indicate that a $1.00 nonprescription remedy would cost at least $1.79 if it had to be prescribed. The only losers, if more medications are made nonprescription, then, are doctors. Why visit a doctor if you can medicate yourself?

The Food and Drug Administration has been keeping dozens of painkillers on the prescription-only list–and no one is quite sure why.

Dr. Sidney Wolfe, director and co-founder of Ralph Nader's Public Citizen Health Research Group, says, "The main legal distinction betweem prescription and over-the-counter drugs is whether the drug can be safely used without the intervention and supervision of a physcian."

But, Tylenol May Not Be Safe!

Wolfe observes, however, "Many people don't consider over-the-counter drugs as drugs." In other words, just because they are available without a doctor's prescription is no guarantee they're safe! Tylenol, for example, the most common brand of acetaminophen, has been associated with kidney disease in several studies.

Tylenol Linked To A Deadly Drug From The Past!

Tylenol is a chemical cousin of phenacetin, a painkiller dating back to 1887 and now banned. Studies make it pretty clear that phenacetin causes fatal kidney disease.

Anthony Temple, of the Tylenol manufacturer McNeil Consumer Products, explained that phenacetin broke down in the body into two chemicals: acetaminophen and something called paraphenetidin. Tylenol does not produce this second chemical, he maintained.

But there is really no proof that this second chemical is what made phenacetin deadly! University of Pennsylvania professor of medicine Dr. Paul D. Stolley says it's "fairly urgent to learn more about acetaminophen. We have a lot of unanswered questions."

Aspirin, Ibuprofen Are No Better!

And aspirin has been linked with gastric bleeding and stomach ulcers. In already ill children, it's found to cause the liver disease Reye's Syndrome.

Even ibuprofen can cause kidney damage, according to studies at Johns Hopkins and at North Carolina's National Institute for Environmental Health Sciences.

Hope For Migraine Sufferers!

So what's a headache sufferer to do? Several natural, non-drug remedies for even severe headaches have come out and are touted not only to work invariably but to have no downside at all.

One is derived from *chrysanthemum parthenium* plants, available in freeze-dried form in capsules at health food stores. It is called feverfew, and just 25 mg twice a day has been shown to prevent migraines or, at least, reduce the pain.

It works by lessening two chemicals in the body that, when over-abundant, are thought to be responsible for the intense headache, nausea, and hyperphotosensitivity of migraines: serotonin, produced by blood platelets, which first constricts and then dilates arteries; and prostaglandin, which is linked to inflammation.

Cayenne Pepper Helps Ease "Cluster" Headaches!

Another natural remedy is called capsaicin. It comes from cayenne pepper, the spicy herb common in Cajun food. Apply capsaicin directly to the painful area—your throbbing temples, for instance.

It will hurt the skin at first, and may burn the eyes or cause the nose to run, as with eating spicy food. But a study in Italy found that repeating the treatment over several days caused the spicy-food reactions to cease and, moreover, significantly cut or, in the majority of cases, completely stopped "cluster" headaches that had previously occurred frequently.

Blocking Nerves That Cause Pain!

Capsaicin works by interfering with the nerves that send pain messages to the brain. The scientific explanation is that it depletes natural compounds called polypeptides, which transmit nerve impulses. Capsaicin can also be diluted in water and sniffed.

Maybe It's Time To Reset
Your Biological Clock!

Finally, a study in California demonstrates that changing your own biological clock can greatly relieve chronic severe headaches. Dr. Lee Kudrow found that either changing your sleep schedule—going to bed and getting up two hours later, say—or exposing yourself to bright fluorescent lights for a few hours every evening at dusk, put an end to chronic headaches after a course of merely two weeks!

The Wonder Tonic: Suma!

Deep in the Amazon jungles of Brazil, natives have been using a natural tonic for all sorts of ailments for, according to some reports, as long as three centuries.

In 1975, the secret was shared with a leading Brazilian herbalist, who introduced the medication to modern civilization. Then, University of Sao Paolo professor of pharmacology Dr. Milton Brazzach did a series of studies confirming that the herbal recipe worked.

He found it was not a cure, but brought significant relief for cancer, diabetes, and gout sufferers, with no undesirable side effects. And doses as low as one gram a day produced basic feelings of well-being.

In the U.S., this Brazilian wonder tonic is now sold as a dietary supplement under the name "Suma." In Brazil, it is known as *para todo*—for everything.

Help For Impotence And PMS!

Indeed, further studies in Japan indicate that Suma is good for impotence, anxiety, and ulcers as well. And Dr. Amanda L. McQuaid, in this country, found that it balances estrogen levels in women, thus providing relief for sufferers of PMS, osteoporosis, and postmenopausal symptoms such as moodiness and low energy levels.

Other studies show benefits to your circulation, cholesterol levels and general healing from injuries.

Suma Is 100% Natural!

Suma seems to work by boosting your immune system. Dr. McQuaid explains, "Suma is an immune-enhancer, fitting into the category of remedies which help us adapt to new stresses and restore natural immune resistance."

Its botanical name is *pfaffia paniculata*, part of the *amaranth* family. It is often thought of as Brazilian ginseng, but it's not really related to ginseng at all.

How It Works!

Among Suma's working ingredients is pfaffic acid, which prevents the spread of various cell disorders. Suma also contains a kind of metal called germanium, which is thought to help fight cancer and facilitate the spread of oxygen throughout the body.

What's more, a number of pfaffocides and other saponins —chemicals derived, essentially, from sugar—help Suma stop diseases already in progress. And the allantoin in Suma, along with other minerals, vitamins, and amino acids, helps accelerate healing.

With Suma, reports say, circulation is improved too, and high cholesterol lowered! This is due to certain hormones in Suma, called sitosterol and sigmasterol, which are said to do wonders for your metabolism.

Now Available In Convenient Packages!

Suma concentrates the natural tonic into convenient 500 mg pills. Two to six tablets a day should do the trick for most everyday ailments.

The Suma extract is made into tablets under strict supervision of the U.S. Food and Drug Administration. Its importers stress that no harm comes to the Brazilian forests from which it is derived. It is picked by hand, and no herb less than seven years old is used.

Because it helps the human body fight illness naturally, it is considered an adaptagen. It gently stimulates normal resistance while, at the same time, working to soften and decrease malignancies.

It helps fight normal bodily wear and tear caused by stress, too, studies attest, and in larger doses has actually been shown to reduce the growth of tumors. It has also been used to fight anemia and bronchitis.

An Ancient Secret
That Could Save Your Life!

And, again, even at higher doses of 10 to 18 grams daily, no side effects were reported.

So, after 300 years, the secret is out. Suma may not only help you feel more rested, confident, and energetic; it may even prolong your life!

Sources Of The Substances Mentioned In This Chapter:

Bio-Oxidative Treatment:
> The International Bio-Oxidative Medical Foundation
> P.O. Box 61767, Dallas, TX 75261
> Phone (817)481-9772

Calcium supplements: CAL-ACID

L&H Vitamins, Inc.	OSTEO HEALTH
38-01 Thirty-fifth Avenue,	Gero Vita International,
Long Island City, NY 11101	Dept. Z101, 2255-B Queen Street East #820,
Phone (800) 221-1152	Toronto, Ontario M4E 1G3, Canada, (800) 825-8482

Candida Guard:
> Gero Vita International,
> Dept. Z101, 2255-B Queen Street East #820,
> Toronto, Ontario M4E 1G3,Canada,
> (800) 825-8482

Cetylpyridinium chloride: Cepacol mouthwash

Domiphen bromide: Scope mouthwash

Feverfew:
> Any health food or vitamin store, or:
> Eclectic Institute, (800) 332-4372, or
> Frontier Cooperative Herbs, (800) 786-1388

Orthophos:
> L&H Vitamins, Inc.
> 38-01 Thirty-fifth Avenue,
> Long Island City, NY 11101
> Phone (800) 221-1152

Phosfood:
> The Vitamin Shoppe
> 4700 Westside Avenue,
> North Bergen, NJ 07047
> Phone (800) 223-1216

Propolis:
> Many health food stores, or:
> Beehive Botanicals
> Route 8, Box 8257,
> Hayward, WI 54843
> Phone (715) 634-4274, or

Sanguinarine: Viadent mouthwash

> Plac-Gard:
> Gero Vita International,
> Dept. Z101,
> 2255-B Queen Street East #820,
> Toronto, Ontario M4E 1G3, Canada,
> (800) 825-8482

Suma:
> Most health food and vitamin stores.

Volatile oils: Listerine mouthwash

7

Prostate Disorders Can Be Prevented And Even Stopped!

In 1990, former President Reagan made a very public announcement that he was undergoing an operation called a prostatectomy — the removal of the prostate gland. The disclosure spawned a lot of jokes and caused anguished expressions from men across the country.

Physicians, on the other hand, applauded the announcement. It finally brought attention to one of the most common men's health problems — prostate disorders. Unfortunately, it also created some popular misconceptions that remain today.

What Is The Prostate?

That's a question every man should be able to answer. The prostate is a walnut sized gland that rests under the bladder and surrounds the urethra, the canal that carries urine and semen through the penis. An accessory gland in the reproductive system, the prostate produces a large portion of a man's seminal fluids.

Because it is so intimately involved in the genito-urinary tract, an enlarged prostate is often the culprit in urinary problems and even sexual

95

dysfunction. The prostate becomes enlarged whenever the blood circulation to it becomes poor or lymphatic fluids get blocked. The expanded prostate begins to tighten around the urethra, which can make urination difficult — even painful.

Who Is Affected?

Let's face it, any problem centering around the genital area seems private at the least and embarrassing at worst. Men with prostate irregularities often fail to come forward for treatment. Many feel guilt or shame, holding the false belief that they may have acted unhealthy or improperly. Some simply ignore the pain.

The truth is that any man over fifty years of age stands a 60% chance of developing an enlarged prostate gland. Besides Ronald Reagan, musician Frank Zappa, Kansas senator Robert Dole, and broadcaster Roone Arledge have publicly admitted needing treatment for prostate disorders.

Although the prostate rarely causes problems for men under fifty, younger men should not ignore it. The gland may begin to enlarge at any age. Prevention should start well before any alarming symptoms appear.

No one knows the cause of every prostate infection, but statistics show that American men are afflicted with prostate disorders more frequently than Asians and Europeans. Black Americans also suffer from prostate cancer more often than do whites.

The Warning Signs!

There are a number of signs that should warn you that you might have a problem with your prostate. The most common symptom is not hard to miss. When the prostate begins to enlarge, it constricts the urethra. Urinating becomes difficult or painful.

Needing to go to the bathroom frequently throughout the night, or having a flow of urine reduced to a trickle are other early signals that it is time for a prostate exam.

In many cases the bathroom problems may seem to resolve themselves without taking any action. It's possible for this to happen, but often the symptoms become more severe.

Infections Of The Prostate!

The most common ailment of the prostate is known as benign prostatic hypertrophy, or BPH. Largely a product of the aging process, BPH refers to the non-cancerous, gradual enlargement of the prostate.

A swollen prostate usually indicates that a man's body is producing lower levels of testosterone than in previous years. Instead, the body begins producing a dangerous substance called dihydrotestosterone. The dihydrotestosterone in turn stimulates an overproduction of prostate cells. The result is a slowly expanding gland.

Research shows that half of American men aged 60 or older have this condition. Some studies, such as the one conducted by Dr. M. Barry in 1990, suggest that the incidence of BPH may be even higher. A swollen prostate should cause concern, but there is little to fear. BPH is rarely life threatening. In fact, some men can and do live comfortably with an enlarged prostate.

Even so it should not be ignored. BPH can cause a great deal of discomfort, and an inflamed prostate may be a sign of something much worse.

Prostatitis!

Another common malady of the prostate is known as prostatitis. Unlike the natural enlargement that happens with BPH, prostatitis is caused by a bacterial infection. Men of any age can contract it.

Prostatitis is an acute inflammation of the prostate. The symptoms are much more severe. The flow of urine can be partially or totally blocked, which often causes urine retention in the bladder. The infected urine can weaken the bladder, or cause urinary infections. In chronic cases, the bacteria can pass into the bladder and spread upward into other vital organs.

Signs that an infection has become advanced are difficulties or irritation during urination, blood in the urine, or pains in the lower back or between the scrotum and rectum. Severe cases need immediate treatment.

Third Most Common Cancer!

Prostate cancer is the third most common cancer found in males. One in eleven American men will develop cancer in their prostate, and it kills more than 30,000 people annually. Studies indicate that prostate cancer is on the rise in the U.S.

For instance, in 1970 research showed that 60 men out of 100,000 were infected with prostate cancer. In 1990, the number increased to 120 out of 100,000. That's a rise of 100%!

Like the other prostate disorders, symptoms occur because of an enlarged prostate. The difference here is that deadly cancerous cells cause the swelling. Warning signs of prostate cancer are the same as for BPH and prostatitis—the biggest reason why you should never ignore painful urine flow.

A digital rectal exam can determine whether or not a prostate is cancerous. A healthy prostate has a firm, rubbery feel to it. Cancer causes it to become stiff like wood. Physicians recommend that every man over forty should have a prostate exam at least once every three years.

Three Billion Dollars
For Prostate Surgery!

Considering the prevalence of BPH, it seems every man will seek treatment for a prostate disorder sooner or later. *The New York Times* reported in 1990 that American men spent over three billion dollars on prostate surgery.

Urologists tend to follow two time-honored paths when combating a prostate problem. The first is to employ a system of "watchful waiting." The second is the more aggressive approach of surgery.

Wait And See?

The prostate generally enlarges very slowly. If the level of discomfort is not very great, some men choose to wait and see if the symptoms improve without treatment. Urine flow often returns to normal levels because men unwittingly adapt to the problem by strengthening their bladder muscles.

Patients should never decide on their own to take this approach. Always consult with a doctor to ensure that symptoms have improved or stabilized. Having a doctor monitor a problem can really pay off. Seventy-five percent of the men who wait a year to put off surgery find that the procedure becomes unnecessary.

Going Under The Knife!

Techniques of today are far better than they were at the turn of the century. In earlier times, castration was the method used to combat BPH. It's no wonder that men get skittish about going to the doctor when they think they have a urinary or genital malfunction.

Presently, surgery is the preferred method for treating prostate disorders. In 1990 alone, doctors performed more than 400,000 prostatectomies. The standard procedure in 95% of the operations performed in the U.S. is called a transurethral resection of the prostate, or TURP.

The TURP is a relatively simple procedure that requires no incisions. It's a bit like scooping out the innards of a sliced melon. A urologist winds a tiny, tube-like instrument called a resectoscope through the penis and up into the urethra. An electrified wire inside the scope scrapes away the excess tissue.

Because the procedure is so unintrusive, a man typically is back on his feet the day after surgery. A catheter is needed to urinate for a few days, but usually is discarded before a patient is discharged from the hospital.

Surgery May Shorten Lifespan!

The TURP procedure has been touted as virtually risk free. That certainly accounts for its popularity with urologists, but some doctors are beginning to seek alternative methods for treating patients with BHP.

When the diagnosis is cancer, surgery is probably unavoidable, but with BHP, a TURP might not be as effective or as risk-free as once believed.

Most reports state that the chance of death following a TURP is a low one percent. Recent federal studies of Medicare patients indicate a slightly higher mortality rate that varies between 3% and 9%. The discrepancy depended upon the hospital.

Dr. John E. Wennberg, an epidemiologist at Dartmouth Medical School in New Hampshire, conducted an independent study in 1990 that produced some surprising results. Urologists believe that early surgical treatment to combat BHP helps patients live longer. The Wennberg research indicated that, rather than help, the preemptive surgery actually lowers life expectancy!

More alarming still, the Wennberg report, published in the Spring 1990 edition of the *New England Journal of Medicine,* showed that TURP patients were more likely to suffer heart attacks than those who chose a different procedure.

Caution: Side Effects!

In addition to these new concerns, the operation does cause some side effects. According to Dr. Herbert Lepor, an associate professor at the Medical College of Wisconsin in Milwaukee, about 6% of patients, or approximately 25,000 in 1990, who had a TURP, suffer from impotency. The cause of impotency is often psychological, however.

A more frequent postoperative problem is retrograde ejaculation, commonly referred to as a dry orgasm. "Patients have the normal sensation of orgasm," says Dr. Lepor, "but they don't have an emission." After the procedure the bladder often fails to close around the urethra properly during ejaculation. The semen shoots back into the bladder rather than out the penis. A man with this condition becomes infertile.

An embarrassing side effect, but one that occurs with less frequency, is incontinence — the inability to control urination. 5% of men who have the operation report incontinence, though the problem usually resolves itself over time.

Surgery itself is not a cure for a prostate that slowly enlarges with age. Even when the procedure is successful, the condition can reoccur. 10% of men who have a TURP need a second operation within five years.

TURP Alternatives!

There are a handful of alternatives to the TURP that offer relief from symptoms of an enlarged prostate. Some have such a short track record that it is impossible to tell what their long term effectiveness may be at this juncture.

A procedure fast gaining in popularity is where surgeons insert a tiny balloon into the urethra to the prostate. They inflate the balloon at high pressure which reopens the clogged passageway. At present the method only works well for patients with advanced BPH symptoms. The drawback is that it seems to offer only temporary relief.

A microwave treatment inserts a wire into the urethra that heats and destroys excess prostate tissue. A similar procedure, used by Terrance R. Malloy, chief urologist at Pennsylvania Hospital in Philadelphia, uses ultrasound to bombard the enlarged prostate. The intense sound waves break away prostate cells which are then sucked away with an aspirator.

Prostate Medications!

Considering the expense of surgery, not to mention the stress factor, patients and doctors have sought a way to treat an enlarged prostate without resorting to an operation. The focus of research was a drug that could counteract the impact of hormones that promoted prostate growth.

Scientists at first concentrated on a drug that blocked the increase of dihydrotestosterone. Unfortunately, the blocking agents also blocked testosterone which caused a loss of libido, impotency, and even breast enlargement—worse conditions than the problem it sought to solve.

A second area of research focused on adrenal hormones, which govern blood pressure and the muscles surrounding the prostate. The first drugs produced in these studies caused debilitating side effects and tumors in laboratory animals during the testing stage.

In 1987, however, Abbott Laboratories, located near Chicago, introduced a drug called Hytrin, a pill used primarily for people with high blood pressure. Called an alpha-blocker by scientists, Hytrin relaxes muscle tissue like the kind found in arteries and the prostate. Early research shows that Hytrin provides immediate relief of many BHP symptoms in about two thirds of the patients who use it.

Although Hytrin was not specifically developed for prostate disorders, physicians can prescribe it for BHP. Patients who use it report good results, though it does cause mild side effects such as dizziness, fatigue, and occasional fainting spells.

The alleged breakthrough in a prostate medication came in 1992 with the introduction of Proscar. Developed by the pharmaceutical giant, Merck & Company, Proscar has received a lot of attention in recent months.

Is Proscar The Answer?

For many men, the response is yes. Officials at Merck estimate that over 100,000 men already take the drug every day. They'll take it for the rest of their lives, if it proves as effective as touted.

Proscar blocks the agents that cause the hormone testosterone to convert into dihydrotestosterone, the catalyst that promotes prostate cell growth. It can't help people with prostate cancer, but its makers claim it can reduce the swelling caused by BHP.

Questions remain about Proscar's effectiveness and its costs. A study published in the October 1992 edition of the *New England Journal of Medicine* compared 300 men with enlarged prostates who took Proscar against a group who took a placebo pill.

The tests showed that Proscar did help relieve some of the symptoms of BHP. The catch was that the drug does not have an impact until a patient takes it for six months to a year.

Further, the research indicated that the improved urine flow increased only by about 17%, compared with the 50% rise afforded patients who choose surgery.

Considering the costs of the drug — about two dollars a pill — Proscar treatment would amount to an outlay of $730 a year. An expensive solution indeed.

Proscar does not, however, bypass the side effects that earlier drugs created. Sexual dysfunction is still a problem. As many as five percent of the sample subjects reported that Proscar lowered the sex drive, the amount of ejaculate, and even caused impotence.

Merck warns that Proscar damages semen and has caused birth defects in laboratory animals. Couples are advised to use contraception when the male takes the drug. It is impossible to determine yet if long-term use causes any other side effects.

Natural Solutions To Old Problems!

It's surprising that so much time and research was spent in producing prescription drugs for prostate disorders. Many doctors believe that natural solutions are the key to solving this age old problem.

There are a number of health problems that seem to affect people in the United States more than in other countries. Nutritionists are beginning to recognize that the reason may be our heavy reliance on processed foods.

Ten Times More Zinc Needed By The Prostate!

Prostate disorders are clearly on the upswing in American men. The aging of the population is a contributing factor, but an often overlooked suspect is the type of foods available. Most store bought items undergo an extensive amount of processing. All this processing destroys a very important ingredient in the male diet —zinc.

Scientists have learned that the prostate uses ten times more of this mineral than any other organ in the body. Zinc picolinate does naturally what drugs like Proscar try to do with chemicals: block the body's production of dihydrotestosterone.

Dr. Earl Mindell, author of the best selling book, *The Vitamin Bible*, writes, "Most zinc in food is lost processing, or never exists in a substantial amount due to nutrient-poor soil."

Further support of this claim comes from Dr. Denham Harman, professor emeritus at the Nebraska School of Medicine and the developer of the free radical theory of aging, who says, "Some 90% of the population consumes a diet deficient in zinc." It's no wonder that prostate disorders are on the rise.

Studies Lend Support!

Two research teams published recent studies that confirm zinc picolinate's contributions to a healthy prostate. Dr. M. Fahim and Dr. J. Harman reported in a government medical journal that zinc was effectively used to reduce prostate enlargement. It also controlled many of the painful symptoms.

A separate investigation by Dr. G.D. Chisholm, published in the *Journal of Steroid Biochemistry*, additionally confirmed the view that zinc picolinate prevented swelling of the prostate. Iron has long been held as a necessary mineral for women's health. These studies indicate that zinc may soon become known as the "man's vitamin."

What To Do?

Men with prostate problems, and those who want to prevent them from occurring, should consider taking zinc supplements. Zinc can provide additional benefits according to observations by Dr. Mindell, "I have even seen success in cases of impotence with a supplement program of B_6 and zinc."

It is important to note that Dr. Mindell suggests a combination of zinc and vitamin B_6. A study by Dr. G.W. Evans published in the *Journal of Nutrition* showed that B_6 (pyridoxine) enhances the body's ability to absorb zinc. The additional supplement ensures that the prostate gets the healthy amount of zinc it needs.

An Old Indian Remedy!

Another natural ingredient that has a long association with prostate health is the saw palmetto berry. Formally known as *Serenoa repens*, this short species of palm tree can be found throughout the lower half of the United States.

The American Indians used it in a number of ways. The seeds were eaten as food, the leaves ground into powder and applied as a poultice for wounds, and the berries were thought to be a mild aphrodisiac, as well as a cure for urinary problems.

Even though it has been listed in pharmacology books for over 80 years, scientists are just now beginning to reexamine *Serenoa's* healthful properties. In 1984, Dr. G. Champault completed a double-blind study that tested *Serenoa's* ability to combat the hormonal imbalance that causes prostate growth.

Champault's report, written in the *British Journal of Pharmacology*, showed that *Serenoa* had a dramatic impact on urine flow for men with BHP symptoms. More interesting still was that *Serenoa* proved much more effective than Proscar. Even so, the FDA has ruled that makers of *Serenoa* extracts may not even hint that it can help men with prostate disorders. Indian medicine men obviously knew something that the FDA doesn't want to believe.

An Accidental Discovery!

During an allergy experiment in 1989, two doctors accidentally discovered that amino acids are important to prostate health. The physicians administered a mixture of three amino acids—glycine, 1-alanine, and glutamic acid—to a group of patients suffering from allergic symptoms. As tests continued, one of the subjects volunteered that his urinary problems had suddenly disappeared.

The disclosure prompted Dr. K.W. Donsbach to initiate a new study. This time the amino acid mixture was given to patients with urinary disorders. Forty men were used in the three month experiment. Twenty received the amino acids, the others were given a placebo. The results were dramatic.

More than 90% of the subjects experienced a reduction in the swelling of the prostate. Almost a third had prostates that returned to normal size. An overwhelming majority spent less time in the bathroom and urinated less frequently, and most reported a much improved urine flow.

Subsequent controlled studies supported Donsbach's results, though there was one caveat. As soon as the subjects stopped taking the supplements, the symptoms slowly returned. The amino acid treatment is a good preventative, but not a cure for BPH.

European Scientists Prove New Substance!

An extract from the bark of an evergreen tree that grows in Madagascar (pygeum africanum) has recently been proven to be the most effective weapon against BHP with no significant side effects.

672 men suffering from prostate disorders were given pygeum or a placebo for six months in double-blind studies at 13 hospitals, three university research hospitals and four other research facilities in France, Germany and Italy. 38 of Europe's most prominent medical scientists supervised the tests and concluded that pygeum corrected the prostate disorders in 66% of the cases studied.

Several prestigeous medical journals published the results of this amazing new medicine which is not available in the United States.

More Alternatives

In the Orient, the powers of ginseng have been lauded for centuries. Indeed, ginseng is cited as a cure for almost any ailment imaginable. Recently, scientists have reported that as far as the prostate is concerned the claims might not be so outrageous.

Dr. W.S. Fahim studied the effect ginseng had on the prostate. His research showed that panax ginseng increased testosterone levels in test animals, while decreasing the size of the prostate. This added confirmation to what many older Oriental men have believed for centuries–that ginseng adds virility, stamina, and an overall improved sex life.

Scandinavians have a secret prostate treatment of their own—bee pollen. *Apis mellifica* pollen has been a common prescription for prostatitis in Europe since the 1960s. A clinical study in 1967 by Dr. Ask-

Upmark, confirmed that the nutrients in the pollen can be a very effective reliever of prostate discomfort.

Recent tests indicate that two other natural products can reduce inflammation of the prostate. *Equisetum* arvense, more commonly known as horsetail, used in tandem with *Hydrangea arborescens*, show a lot of promise as aids to prostate health.

Modern medical research too often resorts to artificial or chemical means to find cures for common ailments. Many times solutions or preventative measures can be found in natural products or vitamin supplements. They are safer, less expensive, and generally come free of any side effects.

If your prostate is giving you problems, it's a good idea to investigate natural solutions before scheduling any surgery or taking prescription medication. Natural products can be the most effective and inexpensive way to improve your health, and promote a better quality of life.

Sources Of The Substances Mentioned In This Chapter:

The following supplements are available in vitamin or health food stores:

Zinc picolinate, B6, pyridoxine, ginseng, *Apis mellifica* pollen (bee pollen), horsetail (Hydrangea), glycine, L-alanine, glutamic acid and saw palmetto (*Serenoa repens*).

One company, Gero Vita International, has combined the proper quantities of each of these into one pill, called "Prostata." To order, write to: Gero Vita International, Dept. Z101, 2255-B Queen Street East #820, Toronto, Ontario M4E 1G3, Canada, or call (800) 825-8482.

8

PMS, Menopause And Osteoporosis–Relief Is Available And Safe!

Often when women are suffering through premenstrual syndrome, or PMS, they get little help from doctors, who tell them it's just another mysterious "female problem." Rather than do the research or take the time to educate themselves about PMS, many doctors prefer to keep their patients–and themselves-in the dark about the causes and available treatments.

Scientists have found that PMS may be caused by the drastic drop in progesterone levels in a woman's body in the week preceding her period. The preeminent scientist on PMS, English physician Katharina Dalton, who coined the term "premenstrual syndrome," first theorized about the role of progesterone. Because of her research, thousands of women with PMS have found relief with progesterone treatments.

Progesterone works to buffer the negative effects that estrogen can have when at elevated levels. During the phase of a woman's cycle when progesterone drops most rapidly, unbuffered levels of estrogen can lead to PMS symptoms, such as low blood sugar, salt and water retention, increased body fat and reduced oxygen levels in the cells.

Avoid Synthetic Progesterone!

Synthetic progesterone is expensive, can only be gotten with a physician's prescription and causes many undesirable side effects. Synthetic progesterone inhibits a woman's production of natural progesterone, which can worsen hormonal imbalance.

Also, some synthetic progesterone is 2,000 times stronger than the natural hormone and can lead to salt and fluid retention and blood sugar imbalances; worse, it can increase the risk of cancer.

Natural Progesterone Is Safe And Effective!

Few doctors are aware of natural progesterone because it can't be patented by pharmaceutical companies, so no drug company is going to launch a multimillion dollar ad campaign to get the word out. But there are natural sources of progesterone that are safe, effective, and inexpensive.

One natural medicine, Ovatrophin, can help raise progesterone levels in a woman who still has her ovaries. It is a glandular medicine made from bovine ovaries. The usual dosage is three pills per day for three weeks and then two pills per day for the next week. The dosage can often be cut down to one pill per day for maintenance after a month of treatment.

Mexican Yam Proven Very Effective And Safe!

A half century ago American scientist Russell Marker discovered a way to extract natural progesterone from wild Mexican yam plants. Traditionally the wild yam had been used by local people to treat menstrual cramps and prevent miscarriage.

Now, the yam extract is available in a blend of aloe vera, vitamin E and vegetable oil, producing a medicinal cream called Pro-Gest

Moisturizing Cream. Multiple studies have found that topical use of the cream significantly raises progesterone levels. As a result, Pro-Gest can be a vital treatment for PMS—and for menopause and osteoporosis too.

Pro-Gest has the extra benefit of being plant-based. Dr. Cynthia Watson, a clinical faculty member at the University of Southern California, has found in her medical practice that botanical hormone supplements are preferable to any other source, because they do not have the side effects of synthetic and animal-based hormones, and they are more easily metabolized.

Pro-Gest Is Easy To Use!

It is generally recommended that Pro-Gest be applied twice daily. In the week before menstruation begins, the cream can be applied up to five times per day if needed. Once menstruation begins, though, the cream should not be used again until bleeding stops.

About 1/4 to 1/2 teaspoon of Pro-Gest should be applied to the abdomen, chest, face or back of the neck. If the appropriate amount of cream is used, it will be absorbed through the skin in three to five minutes. If it disappears in less than two minutes, then more should be used. Once the cream is absorbed, it will change from white to transparent.

By the third month, PMS symptoms should be alleviated, and then Pro-Gest should be used only in the week prior to menstruation. Again, the dosage should be 1/4 to 1/2 teaspoon applied two times per day. More cream can be applied if symptoms are still severe.

While some women choose to use the cream for a few days each month on a long-term basis, many no longer need it after three or four months.

Vitamins Can Provide Relief From PMS!

It is the job of the liver to eliminate excess estrogen, and it needs sufficient amounts of vitamin B_6 (pyridoxine) and magnesium to do this. B_6 is considered by experts to be one of the most important defenses against PMS. Usually women are advised to take a B-complex vitamin daily with 100 mg of B6 and 400 to 800 mg of magnesium.

The *Journal of Reproductive Medicine* reported that many women with PMS are lacking in the minerals and nutrients they need to produce progesterone naturally. For instance, the *Journal of the American College of Nutrition* reported that daily doses of 150 IU of vitamin E can raise progesterone levels.

Keep in mind, though, that high daily dosages of vitamin E can actually LOWER progesterone levels, so keep your dosage below 200 IU per day.

Drawing from the results of animal studies, the journal *Feedstuffs* reported that beta-carotene can increase the synthesis of progesterone. The recommended dosage of beta-carotene is 500 mg per day.

Proof That Pineapple Extract Helps!

A team of scientists reported in *Hawaii Medical Journal* that bromelain, a pineapple extract, aids the production of progesterone, which is needed to balance out excess estrogen. Another study, published in the *American Journal of Obstetrics and Gynecology*, found that bromelain relieves menstrual cramps.

The journal *Recent Advances in Clinical Nutrition* reported that evening primrose oil can also be used to treat PMS because it works much like bromelain in aiding the production of progesterone. The recommended dosage of evening primrose oil is usually 500 mg three times a day.

Pro-Gest Cream Prevents
The Hot Flashes Of Menopause!

Usually when a woman begins menopause, her doctor will prescribe supplemental estrogen because this is the time in her life when estrogen levels naturally begin to decline. Often, though, it is more effective to use supplemental progesterone to treat the symptoms of menopause.

Not only is Pro-Gest Cream good for treating PMS, it can be a real lifesaver for women suffering through the symptoms of menopause.

When hot flashes occur, 1/2 to 3/4 teaspoon of Pro-Gest Cream should be applied topically four times during the hour following the hot flash. At this dosage, symptoms should stop within one week to a couple of months, with individual variations. Once symptoms are under control, a maintenance program can begin with the topical application of 1/4 to 1/2 teaspoon each day.

Extra Benefits Of Natural Progesterone!

Many women experience a drop in their vaginal lubrication after menopause. It has been reported that when applied on the vaginal area, Pro-Gest Cream can increase a woman's natural lubrication.

As an added plus, for some women Pro-Gest Cream has smoothed out wrinkles and faded age spots.

Vitamin E Has Been Proven To Help!

As long ago as 1945, Dr. C.J. Christy published in the *American Journal of Gynecology* the results of his study on menopausal women. Dr. Christy found that when treated with vitamin E, the women experienced significant relief from menopausal symptoms, with no side effects.

A few years later, Dr. H. Ferguson reported in the *Virginia Medical Monthly* the research he did on 66 women with severe symptoms associated with menopause. Dr. Ferguson found that when treated with 15 to 30 IU of vitamin E every day, the women experienced complete relief from their symptoms.

So if the benefits of vitamin E were proven almost 50 years ago, why is the therapy still underused? Because vitamins aren't patentable, and no patent means little profit for pharmaceutical companies, says Dr. R. Passwater, a leading expert on menopause.

Osteoporosis Afflicts 20 Million Older Americans!

Osteoporosis, or brittle bone disease, is a horrible and crippling disease plaguing the nation's elders. A few years ago at the International Symposium on Osteoporosis held in Denmark, a specialist warned, "More women die from osteoporosis-related fractures than from cancer of the breast, cervix and uterus combined, and in the United States hip fracture health care costs up to $10 billion annually, causing 200,000 deaths."

This debilitating disease causes severe weakening of the bones, often leading to a loss in bone mass of as much as 30 to 40%. Millions of fractures occur every year because of this disease. A study carried out in Knox County, Tennessee, found that the number of fractures resulting in hospitalization doubled every five years in people over 50.

Thousands of people break their wrists and suffer collapsed spinal vertebra, a painful and disfiguring problem. But the most devastating injury is the hip fracture: One out of three women and one out of six men after the age of retirement will suffer hip fractures.

Women Most At Risk!

Women most likely to develop osteoporosis are those who don't get much exercise, have small frames, have kidney disease, smoke and drink alcohol, use steroids or thyroid medication, had their ovaries taken out before they were 40 years old, have family members with osteoporosis, or are of Northern European, Latin or Asian background.

For people who suffer hip fractures, often the most devastating part is the loss of independence. Half will never again be able to walk without assistance. Many have no choice but to stay in a convalescent hospital, where they may end up feeling more frail and burdensome.

Profiteering With Estrogen Therapy!

The medical establishment has for years run a one track campaign insisting that all postmenopausal women should receive estrogen therapy for the rest of their lives. And because of this, pharmaceutical companies manufacturing estrogen are raking in the profits hand over fist.

Research has shown that long-term synthetic estrogen use does prevent further bone deterioration. But Dr. Cynthia Watson of the University of Southern California reports that the hormone is really only effective in fighting bone loss during the first five years after menopause. And some researchers are finding that standard estrogen replacement therapy may be helpful in only 25% of the cases.

Most importantly, estrogen CANNOT replace bone that had been lost already before treatment; it merely slows further deterioration.

The Dangers Of Synthetic Estrogen!

Artificially raising the levels of estrogen in postmenopausal women runs against the grain of nature. The body's natural balance is designed for a decrease in the hormone. Disrupting the natural balance can lead to very serious consequences.

Researchers have found that artificially high levels of estrogen can lead to high blood pressure, abnormal blood clotting, diabetes, cancer and liver and gallbladder disease. Women who take estrogen are as much as 14 times more likely than other women to develop uterine cancer.

In fact, even the manufacturers of Premarin, one of the most prescribed estrogen replacement therapies, admit that the drug increases a woman's risk for uterine and breast cancer and can cause a whole host of deleterious side effects, including hair loss, tumors, migraines, depression and worsening of heart disease.

There Are Natural Alternatives To Treat Osteoporosis!

Progesterone derived from plants has been proven to play a vital and unique role in treating osteoporosis. Amazingly, it can reverse the damaging bone loss caused by the disease.

In fact, no treatment that EXCLUDES natural progesterone has been able to improve bone density and strength in people with osteoporosis.

Pro-Gest Cream Helps Regenerate Lost Bone!

Medical researcher Dr. John Lee studied the effects of Pro-Gest Cream when used along with a common treatment plan for osteoporosis. He found that over the course of six months of treatment, bone density increased by up to 10%. When treatment was continued, bone density improved at a rate of 3 to 5% per year until plateauing at the level generally found in healthy 35-year-old women, as reported in the prestigious British medical journal *Lancet*.

Most importantly, Dr. Lee's regimen, which included 100 post-menopausal women aged 38 to 83, improved bone density across the board—regardless of age or time since menopause. This is a critical advantage over an estrogen-only program, because estrogen has been found to help only in the first five years after menopause.

Remarkably, women who began Dr. Lee's study with the most bone deterioration experienced the most improvement over the course of the program. And none of the women in the study suffered bone fractures.

Many of the women in Dr. Lee's program found that their sex drive returned to normal and that they had more energy, more mobility and less aches—with no side effects!

Milk Is Not Enough
To Prevent Osteoporosis!

We all know that children should drink calcium rich milk for strong bones, so the same must go for adults, right? Wrong. Americans drink more milk than anyone else in the world, but we also have the highest occurrence of bone ailments. Obviously, the milk isn't helping.

Dr. N.M. Lewis of the University of Wisconsin Department of Nutritional Sciences studied people on dairy rich diets and found that they excreted the majority of the calcium they consumed.

Worse yet, Dr. R.R. Recker reported in the *American Journal of Clinical Nutrition* that the large amounts of protein and phosphorous in milk cause the body to LOSE more calcium than it gains.

Special Mineral Combination Builds
Healthy Bone!

Calcium supplements alone can't do the job of protecting you from osteoporosis because the mineral can be absorbed into the body only when the stomach produces a healthy level of acid.

Dr. M. Grossman reported in the journal *Gastroenterology* that about 40% of postmenopausal women have extremely low levels of stomach acid. And Dr. R.R. Recker reported in the *American Journal of Clinical Nutrition* that people with low acid levels can absorb only 4% of an oral dosage of calcium carbonate. Healthy people absorb about 22%.

When calcium is taken with other nutrients and minerals, absorption improves. Dr. Recker found that people deficient in stomach acid could absorb calcium citrate at more than 10 times the rate of calcium carbonate.

Researchers have found that special combinations of other important minerals, such as zinc, copper, boron, magnesium, manganese, silicon and even strontium, can help build bone and increase density. Dr. Cynthia

Watson recommends the supplement Osteo Health, which provides many of these necessary nutrients.

Boron Is Key In Fighting Osteoporosis!

Vegetables, kelp, nuts and fruits as easy to find as grapes and apples all contain the vital mineral boron. Nutritional expert Dr. Earl Mindell reports that boron may slow down bone loss in postmenopausal women. Boron's beneficial role is twofold: It helps the body retain dietary calcium, and it can greatly increase the levels of natural estrogen.

Dr. F.H. Nielsen found in his study on boron that deficiencies in the mineral leads to abnormal bone formation. He estimates that people need one to two milligrams of boron daily.

Vitamins Can Help Protect You From Osteoporosis!

The *Journal of the American Geriatrics Society* has published two independent studies finding that people over 65 are commonly deficient in vitamin B_6, vitamin B_{12} and folic acid. These important studies, conducted by Dr. H. Barker and Dr. C. Infante-Rivard, were able to establish a link between low levels of these nutrients and osteoporosis.

Women who have taken birth control pills are particularly at risk because the pill causes vitamin B_6 deficiency. To avoid the health problems—including bone disease—of long-term B_6 deficiency, women taking birth control pills should supplement their diet with at least 50 mg of B_6 per day.

Both vitamins C and K are important for building a strong matrix within bones, and deficiencies can lead to bone disease. A study of patients with osteoporosis found they had vitamin K levels of only 35% of healthy people of the same age. Other studies have found that vitamin K supplements increase bone growth after a fracture and also reduce the amount of calcium excreted in the urine by up to 50%.

Vitamin D is needed to absorb calcium. The level of vitamin D in the elderly tends to be half that of younger people. Dr. R.M. Francis reported in the *New England Journal of Medicine* that vitamin D deficiency can lead to serious bone loss. Although some vitamin D treatments can be expensive and difficult to manage, studies have found that the minerals magnesium and boron can naturally boost levels of the vitamin in the body.

You Can Help Yourself!

Medical problems associated with PMS, menopause and osteoporosis seem very scary and overwhelming—but they don't have to be. You don't need to get an M.D. or pay a lot of money to make yourself healthy. All you need is a little knowledge—which you now have from reading this chapter—and the courage to help yourself. So don't let the pharmaceutical companies pull the wool over your eyes. Stay informed of safe and inexpensive alternative treatments, and you'll be doing yourself and your body the favor of a lifetime.

Sources Of The Medicines Mentioned In This Chapter:

Pro-Gest Cream is made by Professional and Technical Services, Inc., located at 3331 N.E. Sandy Blvd., Portland, OR 97232. To get order for information on ordering, call their main office at 1(800)648-8211 or (503)231-7244.

Ovatrophin is produced by Standard Process Laboratories and can be ordered by contacting the company at 1200 W. Royal Lee Dr., Palmyra, WI 53156. You can also order Ovatrophin through the Vitamin Shoppe at 1 (800) 223-1216 or by contacting a doctor who specializes in nutrition.

Another natural alternative to conventional estrogen replacement therapy is PMSupport which contains natural estrogens. It is available from: Gero Vita International, Dept. Z101, 2255-B Queen Street East #820, Toronto, Ontario M4E 1G3, Canada, or call (800) 825-8482.

9

Enjoy A Healthy Sex Life Even In Old Age!

The desire for sex is one of the strongest of human urges. Few would disagree that feelings of arousal and acting on them with loving partners are among the greatest pleasures of life. Doctors almost unanimously agree that a good sex life is important for good health.

Most images of a sexual nature, whether they appear in advertisements or films, depict young people happily and vigorously enjoying the pleasures of their sexuality. But sex is often on the minds of elderly people too, especially if they aren't performing like they once did.

It's unfortunate, but a general fact of life that as people age the desire wanes, or and sometimes even the apparatus doesn't function at the level it did in youth. Lack of sexual vigor often lowers self esteem and can even affect a person's emotional or psychological well being.

For centuries people have equated sexual virility with good health, strength, and overall vigor. Elderly men or women who remain sexually active seem more youthful. To maintain that edge, people throughout the world have sought sexual stimulants—aphrodisiacs.

Ancients Sought Sex Aids!

Nearly every culture throughout the world claims that one substance or another can work as an aphrodisiac. Whether or not any of these remedies worked, the search for a key to restoring sexual vigor has an incredibly colorful past.

Plants or animal parts that resemble the penis have always found advocates. Ginseng and mandrake roots, for instance, which often appear like human dolls, have long histories as sexual stimulants.

Animals with long or exotic horns naturally received attention. An unfortunate casualty of this belief is the African rhinoceros. The poor creature may become extinct because many people feel that a powder made from its tusk makes a powerful aphrodisiac.

Cooked testicles from animals like the bull, known for its ability to service a herd of cattle, continue to attract adherents who believe that after making a meal of them, a man will procure the prowess of a steer.

Tiger penises, Spanish fly, oysters and even rabbit's feet all have champions who claim these ingredients can unlock dormant sexual desires. For some people they may provide some relief, but modern science has been unable to isolate any curative or stimulating properties in any of these folk remedies.

Contemporary Quackery!

Because sex is such a personal subject, and one that causes people to overreact, miracle cures of the past sometimes created a lot of publicity. Men who sought these quack solutions usually found their wallets a little thinner, and their organs still flagging.

"Is there any quest more universal than the pursuit of sexual vigor?" wrote Kirk Johnson, a reporter with *East West Magazine*. "Our lust for sex is a passion matched only, perhaps, by the eternal pursuit of youth." Too true, as the following stories will attest.

A French Tickler!

The first contemporary impotency cure to receive a lot of attention was espoused by a French physiologist named Charles-Edouard Brown-Sequard in 1889. The seventy-two year old professor was nearing the end of an esteemed medical career. At a lecture before members of the Societe de Biologie, Brown-Sequard announced that he had discovered a formula that restored youth and sexual vigor.

He explained to his audience that for over a year he injected himself with an extract created from the crushed testicles of young dogs and guinea pigs. The mixture had a remarkable effect. He had an increased muscle tone, could work in his lab for hours, but most important, it cured his impotency—an achievement his much younger wife greatly enjoyed.

The announcement caused a sensation. Hordes of elderly Frenchmen rushed out to buy the miracle elixir. Demand was so great that Brown-Sequard could barely fill the orders. Scientists of the day, however, had a different reaction.

Careful study of the mixture revealed that it had no impact on sexual disorders. They derided Brown-Sequard's improvement as a self-created placebo effect. The pandemonium Brown-Sequard created quickly dissipated. He died of a stroke five years later, his once golden reputation tarnished for all time.

More Miracle Cures!

A few years later a Viennese doctor named Eugen Steinach came up with a new treatment for sexual dysfunction. Steinach asserted that sperm production quashed the vigor of youth. In order to regain virility, all a man had to do was keep from losing his sperm. The way to do this, Steinach felt, was through a vasectomy.

Surprisingly, a number of men stepped up for the cure. Luckily the operation did not cause any damaging side effects, though it also didn't work as advertised. Modern vasectomy patients can attest to that.

An American Gets Into The Act!

One of the more bizarre yet long-lived impotency cures was invented by a North Carolina drifter named John Brinkley. In 1917, Brinkley, by then calling himself a doctor, operated out of a small practice in Milford, Kansas.

His first patient was a farmer complaining of impotency. In treating the poor man's problem, Brinkley grafted a piece of goat gonad onto the farmer's testicles. A few weeks later the man returned, reporting that he was back in service. It was no joke. Within a year the man sired a son.

Though the scientific community considered the operation an outrage, the publicity brought Brinkley thousands of patients. He stayed in business and out of trouble until 1930 when his medical license was revoked. Assistants continued to perform transplants until 1941, when Brinkley officially retired.

Sex And Happiness!

These miracle potions and operations may seem funny to people who have a healthy sex life, but for those suffering through a bout of impotence it's a serious matter.

The American Psychiatric Association reports that sexual dysfunction is a growing problem in America today. Indeed, studies indicate that one in four persons has some sexual disorder. Masters and Johnson, the noted sex researchers, admit that solving impotency is a major source of "anguish and frustration" for men.

On the other hand, a healthy sex life has many rewards, the least of which are physical. A recent article in the *San Francisco Chronicle-Examiner* by the Rev. Andrew M. Greeley, a professor of sociology at the University of Chicago, claimed that happiness and a good sex life go hand in hand.

The article described the results of a sexuality experiment Greeley conducted between 1988 and 1991. Over 5,700 subjects participated in the test. According to Greeley's data, the happiest people in America are married couples who continue to have sex regularly after age 60.

The Greeley statistics may startle some, but shouldn't. In the Greeley sample, 37% of married people over 60 reported that they have sex at least once a week. A randy 16% claimed they made love at least twice or more. The sexually active aged subjects also tended to rate their lives as happier and more exciting than those whose sex lives were non-existent.

Considering the age and experience of the over 60 crowd, it should come as no surprise that couples who continue to have sex consider their mates great lovers. Indeed, experimentation becomes a major part of the act. The bedroom is not always the favored locale for a tryst. "One-third swam nude together; one-third showered together; one-half enjoyed extended sexual play," wrote Greeley.

It's obvious that satisfying sex over 60 is more than just a dream. But the question for many persists: What to do if the machinery doesn't work like it used to?

Male Sexual Disorders!

Some sexual dysfunction in men can be traced directly to the prostate gland. The gradual enlargement of the prostate is largely a function of the aging process. Besides the more familiar urinary tract disorders, a swollen prostate can make an erection difficult or impossible. The prostate needs specific medication and care to ensure it and your sex life stay healthy. (See chapter 7.)

Aging affects many parts of the body and the erectile tissue of the penis is no exception. As men get older these tissues tend to lose their strength. The result means less firm erections or none at all. That's hardly new information. The centuries old pursuit for the perfect aphrodisiac lends plenty of testimony.

The difference today is that science is beginning to find some answers. Hormones, it should come as no surprise, play a pivotal role. The testosterone level in men shifts at age 18, and again around age 45. The body simply doesn't make as much of it as in previous years. The decrease in testosterone levels makes men tire more easily, reduces muscle tone, and in extreme cases can diminish the sex drive as well as the ability to have an erection.

Women And Testosterone!

Testosterone is important for women too. Most people think of estrogen as the primary female hormone. There's no question that it is, but scientists are just realizing that when it comes to the sex act, testosterone is essential.

"Women with higher testosterone levels have more sex, increased libido, more orgasms and tighter bonds with their mates," reports Dr. Julian Whitaker, editor of *Health and Healing*, a medical newsletter.

Testosterone stimulates the erectile tissue in the female's clitoris in much the same manner that it does the male's penis. It also causes the secretions that help lubricate the vagina. Both of these activities promote arousal for women.

People may wonder that if it's just a problem of low testosterone, why not just give everyone an artificial boost of it. It seems a good suggestion, but unfortunately human body chemistry doesn't respond to that simple a treatment, and synthetic hormones often produce debilitating side effects. Some natural products, however, show promise that they can do what chemicals cannot.

Feeling Your Oats!

Oats have a long history as a folk remedy for an ailing libido. The ancient Greeks were perhaps the first to associate the grain with sex. A sheaf of oats almost always accompanied any depiction of Eros, the Greek god of passion.

The Romans, who borrowed much of their culture from the Greeks, also picked up on the connection. Steaming bowls of oats was the preferred nourishment that attendants would serve to revelers following an afternoon of orgiastic partying.

Perhaps that's why today the phrase "feeling your oats" is considered a connotation for sexual vigor. But most people feel that anyone who believes that oats can help with a sagging libido is falling for an old wives tale. Recent research indicates that maybe the ancients knew more than anyone thought.

An Accidental Rediscovery!

Chinese farmer, Lee Zhang, was a practical man. In addition to growing grains and vegetables typical to most farms, Zhang raised carp in a pond on his property to trade at his local market. The colorful fish also served as emergency rations for his own family when money was tight.

Feeling his son needed to help out more with the day to day chores of the farm, Zhang asked the boy to start feeding the carp before he went off to school. The boy did as he was told and began giving them food from a bag that was stored in the barn.

After a few weeks the boy ran out of food and dutifully told Zhang that they needed to buy some more. Zhang was surprised. He knew the feed supply should have lasted much longer. After investigating, Zhang saw that the bag holding the carp feed was still full. A bag that once held green oats, however, was now empty. His son had fed the carp the wrong food.

Zhang, fearing the worst, immediately checked up on the fish. He was shocked at what he saw. The carp obviously enjoyed their new diet. Hundreds of baby carp swam around in the now crowded pool. Even more, the older carp seemed much livelier and healthy—very unusual for a fish that is normally a lazy breeder. Zhang concluded that the green oats somehow caused the fish to mate much more aggressively.

During trips to the market, Zhang mentioned the story of the miracle carp to his fellow farmers. Word spread of the amazing discovery. The tale eventually caught the ears of researchers who decided to test the oats for themselves.

Scientific Documentation!

Chinese scientists first examined Zhang's carp to see if the story had any validity. They found that various hormone levels in the fish were more than one-third above the norm.

Next they obtained a quantity of the oat mixture to see if they could duplicate the effects in humans. The green oats, along with an amount of a stinging nettle, were ground up into powder and stirred together with water to form a broth.

The Chinese researchers conducted an unofficial experiment by consuming the strange cocktail themselves. The results were surprising. All the scientists reported having more energy. They also noticed that they had much firmer and larger erections than ever.

What Was In That Feedbag?

That's what scientists wanted to know. The oats were not the typical farm brand but a similar strain known as *Avena sativa*. Not an unusual variety, but it was quickly learned that only a fresh batch proved capable of working its magic.

The stimulating qualities of *Avena sativa* were noted as early as two centuries ago by German physicians, who wrote about its positive affects in a pharmacopoeia of the time. A common medicine in folk remedies, oats allegedly cure allergies, eczema, and circulatory and digestive problems.

Added to the oats were a few grains of a stinging nettle known formally as *Urtica dioica*. Another therapeutic plant, *Urtica dioica* has a history of use as an aid for a host of problems, ranging from urinary tract disorders to a cure for anemia.

Even though researchers learned what was in the grain, they were unable to reproduce the original results. Oats alone did nothing; the same was true with a pure nettle extract. For some unexplained reason, the aphrodisiac-like properties only seemed to work when just the right amount of the two grains was added to water.

Further Tests Lend Support!

Academics became skeptical of the extract's powers. New studies focused upon whether or not a measured batch of the mixture truly worked as an aphrodisiac. The Chinese themselves initiated a more valid double-blind experiment a year after its initial discovery.

In it, nearly two hundred men took a stabilized formula of the mixture for several weeks. An astounding 90% of the sample subjects reported that it increased their desire to have sex, and even claimed it improved their performance.

A Hungarian scientist, Dr. Robert Frankl of Budapest University, conducted an independent study in 1984. Twelve male subjects consumed the mixture for several weeks. Dr. Frankl confirmed that the formula helped the men increase their aerobic power and muscle strength. It also increased the testosterone levels of the subjects.

Scientists at the University of Texas studied the extract's effect on horses. Tests verified that it was an effective energy stimulant, and also improved the animal's endurance.

A similar test that used humans as subjects was developed by researchers at the College of Medicine of Northwestern Ohio University. Here, the data was more conclusive. Experiments showed that the nettle and oat mixture helped sexually dysfunctional men develop and sustain an erection. The blood hormone levels of these men markedly increased by 30%.

More Direct Confirmation!

All of these experiments eventually caught the eye of scientists at the Institute for Advanced Study of Human Sexuality, a nonprofit research organization based in San Francisco.

Researchers at the Institute wanted to determine whether or not the nettle-oat extract actually produced any sexual benefits. The results of a six week double blind study using 40 subjects were impressively in favor of the nettle-oat extract.

Using urine samples as an indicator, researchers confirmed that the testosterone levels of men and women participating in the experiment increased an average of 105%. Men suffering from impotency reported they could now perform. Women who claimed they had little or no desire for sex felt pangs of sexual excitement for the first time in years.

Testimony Says It All!

Testimony of the participants lent further support for *Avena sativa's* usefulness for men and women. A 28-year-old woman said she "felt better, more intense orgasms," and had "more sexual dreams."

A 25-year-old female subject felt the mixture really helped stimulate her sense of touch. "You are supersensitive to touch, sexual and nonsexual, especially in your mouth," she reported. "You just want to be all tangled up and real intense."

The report raved about the formula's impact on men. "The overall effect for the men who reported improvement can be summarized as a generalized sense of well-being with an increased ability to function sexually." Most men claimed that the stimulation they felt was "reminiscent of their youth."

The most dramatic reports came during a live taping of the syndicated *Geraldo* TV program. The host, Geraldo Rivera, interviewed Loretta

Haroian, Dean of Professional Studies at the Institute, along with several people who took part in the experiment.

Ray McIlvenna, a 68 year old male participant in the study, provided the show's greatest moment when he announced that after taking the formula his erections became "larger than ever in my life." Geraldo's reaction: "Well, God bless."

More Experiments To Come!

Researchers at the Institute for Advanced Study of Human Sexuality recognize that there is still much to learn about *Avena sativa*. "We will continue," say the Institute's administrators, "to investigate and supervise the research of physicians who are willing to hold the scientific hypothesis that this particular extract of oats or some derivative thereof can restore sexual vigor and enhance the sexual experience of men and women."

More Natural Alternatives!

The bark of the *Corynanthe yohimbe*, a tree found in Cameroon, produces a potent natural drug that many African tribesmen consider a true aphrodisiac. The drug became popular with European sailors during the Renaissance, who learned of its powers from the natives with whom they traded.

Four recent experiments by medical research teams show that yohimbine, the drug made from the tree's bark, may possess genuine aphrodisiacal properties. The results are almost as dramatic as those attributed to green oats.

In 1984 a team of researchers at Stanford University led by Dr. Julian Davidson observed the effect yohimbine had on the sexual activity of rats. A group of rats were rated as sexually active, celibate, or impotent.

After giving them all injections of yohimbine, the scientists observed that the normal male rats mounted the females up to 45 times in a fifteen minute period—twice what would have been normal. Almost half of the sexually inactive rats regained interest in sex and started copulating.

Dr. Alvaro Morales, a urologist at Queens University Hospital in Canada, performed an experiment similar to Davidson's in 1987. The difference was that Morales used 23 impotent men. Ten of the subjects reported some improvement, while six claimed they underwent complete recoveries.

Two later studies supported the Morales results. Yohimbine clearly showed some "modest effectiveness" in combating impotence. A report written by Reid and colleagues in the *Lancet* announced that yohimbine "seems to be as effective as sex and marital therapy for restoring sexual functioning."

An Argentine Aphrodisiac!

In South America, the bark from the *Aspidosperma quebracho*, a hardwood tree in the dogbane family, has a similar reputation. The drug quebracho has an equivalent chemistry to yohimbine, so it should be no surprise that the sexual properties are nearly identical.

Physicians have learned that the blood flow that causes the penis to swell is controlled by the release of the enzyme norepinephrine. Yohimbine and quebracho have proven effective as sexual stimulants because they impact the sympathetic nervous system—which regulates norepinephrine flow. The upshot of all these chemical reactions is more frequent erections.

The Sweet Potato!

The Mexican yam, has gained a lot of recent attention as a possible sexual invigorator. Although far from demonstrated fact, studies suggest that nutrients in the yam can help prevent sexual disorders, and revive a dormant libido.

Mexican yams produce Mother Nature's finest organic steroids. Like the chemical enhancers professional athletes use, steroids help the body increase its muscle mass and recuperative powers. Artificial steroids produce the side effect of reducing the libido. Natural steroids, however, improve it.

The active ingredient in natural steroids is the hormone DHEA (dehydroepiandrosterone). DHEA has many health benefits. It stabilizes blood sugar levels which have shown to decrease sexual ability; and it stimulates the body's immune system, which helps to reinvigorate a number of bodily functions—sexual and nonsexual.

Horny Goat Weed!

Another extract that has shown some efficacy as an aphrodisiac is the humorously named horny goat weed. Daniel Reid, author of *Chinese Herbal Medicine*, writes that horny goat weed increases "sperm count and semen density" in men. Tests also show that it enhances blood circulation, particularly in thin capillaries like those found in the penis.

Sources Of Substances Mentioned In This Chapter:

Two vitamin companies have developed *Avena sativa* and nettle extracts in powder form. Gero Vita International produces SEXATIVA. In addition to the nettle and oat mixture, SEXATIVA also contains zinc, glycine and boron. All of these ingredients have proven effective in helping with sexual disorders. Write to Gero Vita International, Dept. Z101, 2255-B Queen Street East #820, Toronto, Ontario M4E 1G3, Canada, or call (800) 825-8482.

The second product is called EXSATIVA, and is carried by some health food stores. It only contains nettles and oats.

The following are readily available in vitamin and health food stores. Ask sales people to show you samples of horny goat weed, yohimbine or quebacho.

Gero Vita International also produces a querbarcho bark supplement called Mood Elevator. Their address is Dept. Z101, 2255-B Queen Street East #820, Toronto, Ontario M4E 1G3, Canada, or call (800) 825-8482.

DHEA may be available from: Belmar Pharmacy, 8015 W. Almeda Ave., Suite 100, Lakewood, CO 80226, 1-800-525-9473; or College Pharmacy, 833 N. Tejon St., Colorado Springs, CO 80903, 1-800-748-2263.

Vita Potencia, made by Gero Vita International, contains naturally-occuring DHEA from Mexican wild yam.

10

To Eliminate Fatigue And Have More Energy, Your Body Needs Racing Fuel!

As you age, your body becomes less efficient at producing some essential nutrients. Some of the metabolic processes also slow down. Each year your body tends to work a little bit harder to maintain itself. This natural aging process is a big factor contributing to fatigue.

Even though there are many things tiring us, we now know that there are also many ways in which we can counteract the effects of stress, aging and environmental toxins.

Famous athletes today have the best scientific help available to assist them in achieving optimal performance. Literally hundreds of tests of various foods and nutrients have been done on athletes to determine what nutritional supplements make for peak performance of mind and body. Now that information is also available to you.

The Vitality Vitamins!

It is generally agreed that the B vitamins are helpful for stress. Two B vitamins are specificly for enhancing energy. The first is pantothenic acid, also known as B_5.

In a recent double blind study, reported by Dr. D. Litoff in *Medicine and Science in Sports and Exercise*, well-trained distance runners were given pantothenic acid daily for two weeks. These athletes outperformed the athletes who received placebos. The runners who took the pantothenic acid used 8% less oxygen and had nearly 17% less lactic acid buildup than the placebo group—quite a significant difference.

The other important B vitamin is para-aminobenzoic acid (PABA), essential to the body for the breakdown and utilization of proteins and in the formation of blood cells. Dr. Robert Atkins, author of *Dr. Atkin's Superenergy Diet*, recommends para-aminobenzoic acid for alleviating fatigue and achieving optimal energy.

Minerals That Matter!

The two minerals that make a difference in energy levels are magnesium and potassium. Magnesium and potassium are involved in just about every major biologic process, including the production of nucleic acids and protein, the metabolism of glucose and the release of cellular energy. They are also necessary for muscle contraction, nerve conduction, the beating of the heart and regulation of vascular tone.

Deficiency of one or both of these important minerals can lead to high susceptibility to fatigue. In a study of individuals diagnosed with chronic fatigue syndrome (CFS)—sometimes called the "Yuppie Flu" or Epstein-Barr—it was found that all participants diagnosed with CFS had abnormally low levels of magnesium in their blood. In the double blind study, those who received magnesium sulfate injections responded with increased energy, decreased pain and improved emotional states in compared to those who received the placebos.

Other studies in Sweden on well-conditioned athletes found that when the athletes took potassium-magnesium aspartate prior to an exercise stress test they showed an astounding 50% increase in their endurance.

Immune Enhancers Boost Energy!

With thousands of new cases of CFS appearing each month, medical researchers have been investigating the cause of this mysterious disease which can leave its victims debilitated by fatigue for months or years. The prevailing theory at this time is that CFS is related to an imbalance in the immune system and that less severe cases of fatigue can also be related to immune weakness.

Studies have shown that CFS weakens the immune response of a type of lymphocyte (white blood cell) called a natural killer cell, but have also found that there is a supplement that boosts the production of these white cells. These natural substances, discovered by Japanese researchers in 1922, are alkylglycerols found in high concentration in shark liver oil.

Another substance, N,N-Dimethlyglcine (DMG), based on the amino acid, glycine, is also a powerful immune enhancer. In an interesting double blind study, all participants were injected with pneumonia antibodies. Participants given DMG had a higher antibody count in their blood than did participants receiving the placebo.

Several Japanese medical studies have shown that a protein-rich substance found in some algae, Phycotene (phycocyanin), assists in the replacement of leukocytes—essential to proper immune function.

Another powerful immune stimulator is Echinacea. Echinacea was one of the most popular medicinal plants in the U.S. in the 1800s, and recently it has attracted renewed interest. Commonly known as cone-flower, Echinacea has natural antiviral properties and is helpful as well in combating bacterial and fungal infections.

When all of the supplements above are combined, the result is a strong immune system—a robust defender against CFS and less virulent causes of fatigue. The previously mentioned immune enhancers are now available in a product called Immune Focus.

A Secret From The Brazilian Rain Forest!

From the natural cornucopia of the Brazilian rain forest comes Suma, an herb that helps the body adjust to stress. Suma has been reported by Dr. Paul Lee, director of the American College of the Healing Arts, to combat fatigue, prevent colds and flus, speed healing, regulate blood sugar and stimulate sex drive. Dr. Michael Tierra, author of *The Way of Herbs*, reports that his most consistent use of Suma has been in the treatment of chronic fatigue and low energy conditions.

Suma, contains substantial vitamin A, C and germanium—a known immune enhancer. It also is rich in two plant hormones, sitosterol and stig-masterol, which prevent cholesterol absorption and improve blood circulation. Studies have shown Suma to increase both energy and strength while at the same time triggering the body to find its own unique state of balance.

Another Secret From The Same Forest!

Yet another powerful energy-enhancing plant makes its home in the Brazilian rain forest. This one is *Paullina cupana*—known as guarana by the natives. Used by the Brazilians for hundreds of years, the herb, served in tea form, was introduced to European explorers who brought it back to their homelands. Today, it is consumed in liquid form to combat fatigue, increase alertness and decrease hunger.

Although *Paullina cupana* does contain caffeine and tannin, it has several other active ingredients, according to Dr. L. Grieve "It is a gentle excitant, useful for the relief of fatigue or exertion", Grieve explained. Most users report experiencing increased energy and decreased fatigue without the typical "letdown" of other stimulants.

A Wonder Of The Orient!

In China the extracts of the Ginkgo leaves have been used for more than 5,000 years for the treatment of disorders of the heart and lungs. It is widely used today in the Ayurvedic medicine of India and in Mexico and Europe. Over the last few years 34 major studies have been published concerning the healing powers of *Gingko biloba*.

Because *Ginkgo biloba* increases oxygenation of brain tissue, it has been shown to be especially helpful for anyone suffering from decreased blood flow to the brain. A double blind study of elderly participants reported by Dr. Bauer in *Arzneimittel-Forschung/Drug Research* noted improved mental performance in those who ingested the extract over an extended period of time. Dr. Schafler conducted another double blind study on healthy young men subjected experimentally to conditions of low oxygen. He reported, in the same medical journal, that the neurologic responses of the participants receiving the extract were significantly better than those ingesting the placebo.

Other mechanisms of action of Ginkgo include the prevention and repair of oxygen free radical damage to the brain, the increase of nerve transmission and the enhancement of the brain's glucose metabolism.

The mechanism for increasing mental alertness appears to be related to the ability of Gingko to change brain wave frequency. Dr. Pelton in his book, *Mind Food and Smart Pills*, describes a double blind study in which participants were attached to EEG monitors. Those taking the extract exhibited increased alpha brain waves—the waves associated with a relaxed, but alert and clearly focused mind—in comparison to those taking the placebos.

Stimulates Cells To Make More Energy!

Adenosine triphosphate (ATP) stores energy in the body's cells, and its production is stimulated by allantoin. When ATP levels are low you feel sluggish and tired. Many people do not have sufficient allantoin in their diets for efficient ATP production, partially due to the eating of refined grains which lose allantoin during processing.

Symphytum, commonly known as comfrey, is a rich source of allantoin as well as vitamins A and C, potassium, magnesium, phosphorous, iron, sulfur, copper, zinc, 18 amino acids and protein. Your cells will thank you for adding comfrey to your diet.

The Energizing Wild Yam!

Dehydroepiandrosterone (DHEA) is produced by the adrenal glands and is also found in the Mexican wild yam. As you grow older your blood levels of DHEA steadily decline, as does your energy level.

Recent research by Dr.Barrett-Conner published in the *New England Journal of Medicine* provides interesting evidence in this regard. The study followed 242 men over an extended period of time. The findings showed that not only did DHEA levels decrease with age, but that those with histories of heart disease had particularly low levels. In general, there was an increased risk of death from any cause associated with lower levels of DHEA.

In another study, Alzheimer patients were found to have DHEA blood levels that were 48% lower than age-matched controls. Yet the non-Alzheimer patients, in turn, had levels 50% lower than a healthy, younger group.

In yet another double-blind experiment by Dr. Vincent P. Calabrese of the Medical College of Virginia show a positive relationship between the use of DHEA and the relief of fatigue. In this study 64% of the multiple sclerosis patients receiving DHEA reported a significant reduction in fatigue and improved stamina.

Makes People Look 15 Years Younger!

Ribonucleic acid (RNA) builds protein in the body. As you age there is an increasing probability of shortages and breakdowns in nucleic acid, leading to errors in RNA and protein synthesis.

Dr. Benjamin Frank explained in his book, *Nucleic Acid Nutritional Therapy*, that dietary nucleic acids are essential for optimal health. He noted that individuals who take RNA supplements on a regular basis appear 5 to 15 years younger than their actual age.

Dr. Milton Fried reports many beneficial results for individuals taking RNA supplements, including improved memory, less fatigue upon physical exertion, improved tolerance of extremes in temperature, better near vision, enhanced immunity and tighter, more radiant skin.

More Vitality And Faster Healing!

Another supplement, coenzyme Q10, plays an important catalytic role in the process of cellular energy production. Dr. Peter Mitchel and Dr. Karl Folkers, who discovered its vital role, were awarded the Nobel Prize and the Priestly Medal of Honor, respectively.

Recent studies, including those conducted by researchers at the Institute for Bio-Medical Research at the University of Texas and at the Methodist Hospital in Indianapolis, have shown that CoQ10 has improved heart muscle metabolism and is effective in the treatment of congestive heart failure and coronary insufficiency.

It has been found that most people over the age of 50, and individuals with heart disease, cancer, gum disease or who are obese have low levels of CoQ10. The addition of CoQ10 to their diets has resulted in increased vitality, faster healing, improved immunity, strengthening of the heart and normalization of blood pressure.

The Energetic Effect Of Germanium!

Another important supplement is germanium. A biologically active trace element, germanium was introduced to the public by Dr. Kazuhiko Asai, who described the work at his clinic in his book, *Miracle Cure: Organic Germanium.*

Since GE-132 increases cellular oxygen uptake, it improves circulation and cardiovascular functioning. It also normalizes high blood pressure and cholesterol. Its energetic effect has been most noticeable in middle aged to elderly sedentary individuals, according to Dr. Rinchardt.

A paper presented at the Osaka International Symposium reported that GE-132 intake resulted in the alleviation of joint pains and morning stiffness, while Russian researchers shared findings at a recent international AIDS conference that GE-132 inhibits HIV reproduction in test tube studies.

RNA. CoQ10 and GE-132 are now available in one combined product, RNA Plus.

Sources Of Substances Mentioned In This Chapter:

The following supplements mentioned in the foregoing are available from health food or vitamin stores: Para-aminobenzoic acid (PABA), panothenic acid, potassium-magnesium aspartate, ginkgo biloba, *Symphytum* (comfrey), RNA supplements, *Echinacea*, shark liver oil, DMG, Suma and *Paullina cupana* (guarana).

A combination of many of these are available in Immune Focus (containing shark liver oil, DMG, phycotene and *Echinacea*) and in RNA Plus (containing RNA, coenzyme Q10 and germanium). These two combination products are available from Gero Vita International, Dept. Z101, 2255-B Queen Street East #820, Toronto, Ontario M4E 1G3, Canada, or call (800) 825-8482.

DHEA may be available from: Belmar Pharmacy, 8015 W. Alameda Ave., Suite 100, Lakewood, CO 80226 or call (800) 525-9473.

Vita Potencia, made by Gero Vita International, contains naturally-occuring DHEA from Mexican wild yam.

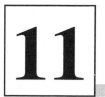

Skin Care Takes Giant Leap Forward!

We'll all have problems with our skin at some point or another. We may not remember the diaper rash of our cradle years, but few of us can forget acne, which many of us suffered at least some degree in our teen years. And those of us who are not already experiencing the mid-adult years can look forward to age spots, wrinkles, and permanent bags or circles under our eyes as our skin begins to show the weariness of age.

The skin of an average-size adult will cover about 20 square feet if laid out flat, writes Dr. D. Chapman in *The Biochemical Journal*. The largest organ of our bodies is, as a matter of fact, our skin. It is a complex organ with three primary functions: regulating body temperature, protection, and acting as a tactile organ (i.e., giving us our sense of touch).

Each of these layer of skin is susceptible to disease and photoaging (sun damage), wrinkling, yellowing, and mottling or splotching.

Several Alternative Remedies
Are Available For Skin Problems!

Beauty may be only as deep as this thin organ, but many of us are concerned about its health and appearance. Fortunately, relief is available from several little known products for such problems as acne, scars, painful or itchy skin diseases, varicose veins and especially our inevitable wrinkles.

Some of these wrinkle fighting health products offer additional anti-aging benefits, which include help for the fight against gray or thinning hair, brittle nails and age spots. Others can help reduce cellulite or scars as well!

Beware Of Premature Skin Aging Villains!

Wrinkles and other signs of aging skin can be caused or enhanced by several culprits. Stress, a lack of sleep or exercise, illness, smoking, poor nutrition and pollution are some of these, but one of the worst premature skin-aging villains is the sun, according to Dr. Allen Lassus, a researcher in the Department of Dermatology at University Central Hospital in Helsinki, Finland.

Dr. Attila Dahlgren was a child prodigy who received his medical degree at the young age of 25. Working with his associate Manuel Haipern, a heart and aging specialist from the University of Lisbon, Dr. Dahlgren studied the damaged, wrinkled skin of patients aged 20 through 80. He discovered that ultraviolet (UV) radiation from the sun often causes heliodermatitis, a low-grade inflammation in the lower two layers of skin. If we continually expose ourselves to UV rays, Dr. Dahigren explained, the heliodermatitis becomes chronic.

Chronic heliodermatitis congests the skin's capillaries. Since capillaries feed nutrients from the blood to the skin's membranes, congested capillaries equal starved skin. Protein fibers that hold the skin together, keeping it smooth and healthy, break down when the skin becomes mal-nourished.

This fiber breakdown, in turn, causes the skin to lose its ability to retain moisture. The visible result is that the drier the skin gets, the deeper its creases become.

Out Of The Dentist Office And Into Your Cosmetic Case!

We all reach that day when our laugh lines show even when we're not laughing. Many of us consider face lifts at this time. But there are several simpler ways to ease creases and other signs of aging than facing the pain and expense of plastic surgery.

Your dentist has one key to unlock youth's door: procaine, also known as Novocain. The positive results of procaine on such aging signs as wrinkling, hair loss and graying, and hardened tissues have been well documented. Between 1930 and 1951, in fact, more than 165 studies were published revealing procaine's benefits in the fight to combat aging, according to an article in *Anti-Aging News*.

The components of procaine are available in a chemical free anti-aging skin cream called Gero Vita GH3 Mature Skin Revitalizer.

In the periodical *Cosmetics & Toiletries*, Dr. J.A. Hayward states that the famed Geriatric Institute of Romania used a similar cream as its primary form of treatment for wrinkles. Since treatments could cost $10,000 a week or more, the Institute catered only to those who could afford it, including celebrities such as Elizabeth Taylor, Kirk Douglas, Aristotle Onassis, Marlene Dietrich and Cary Grant.

Procaine Is Rich In Nutrients!

Procaine is created in the laboratory by bonding two vitamin nutrients with gigantic names: para-aminobenzoic acid (PABA) and diethylaminoethanol (DEAE).

When taken into the human body, according to Dr. D. Chapman in *The Biochemical Journal*, procaine is broken down into PABA and DEAE as well as an additional nutrient by-product, dimethylaminoethanol (DMAE). DEAE and DMAE enhance tissue circulation and stimulate the production of phosphatidylcholine, one of the building blocks of cellular membranes. Dr. Chapman states that "cellular membrane degradation" is one of the primary causes of aging.

PABA is a B vitamin that helps form metabolizing proteins and healthy blood cells. It also works as an aid to keep hair, glands and intestines inoptimum condition.

Mature Skin Revitalizer Gives Skin Important Nutrients!

Mature Skin Revitalizer cream mixes PABA, DEAE and DMAE with liposomes—tiny spheres made from various of lipids, expIains Dr. Ronald DiSalvo, research director for Paul Mitchell Cosmetics and one of the developers of the cream. (Lipids are organic substances that store reserve energy in the body.) "When applied topically, these liposomes are able to penetrate and reach aging skin tissue," DiSalvo says.

In order to minimize contamination, Gero Vita GH3 Mature Skin Revitalizer is not sold in jars; rather, it is distributed in bottles with special non-contaminating applicators. The reason for this is simple: creams can lose their potency when they come in contact with dirt, oils and emollients from fingers. Mature Skin Revitalizer's non-contaminating applicator ensures that remaining cream is never touched when a dose is applied to the skin. This maintains the cream's potency.

An Anti-aging Cream That Fades Scars!

Another non-prescription cream can help heal sun damaged skin, fade age spots and other blemishes, and diminish small wrinkles; and in addition to such anti-aging qualities, it helps fade scars as well! Skin Secrets Glycolic Renewal is the name of the cream. Its active ingredient is a natural derivative of sugar cane: glycolic acid.

Dr. James Leyden, a professor of dermatology at the University of Pennsylvania, tested 40 people with creams containing glycolic acid. "We saw improvements in all of the test subjects," he attested. "The thin wrinkles disappeared and their skin was smoother and fresher looking."

Removes Dead Cells To Let Fresh Cells Take Over!

Glycolic acid has properties that help to slough away dead cells from the skin's surface. This gives new cells a chance to emerge and show themselves off in the form of smoother, younger looking skin.

The application of creams containing glycolic acid will generally bring about noticeable skin improvements within three to seven days. Daily use of such products over a period of six to twelve months can mean dramatic improvements—diminishing deep skin creases and virtually eliminating fine lines.

Former Miss America Loves It!

Susan Akin—Miss America of 1986—testified glowingly about the effects of Skin Secrets Glycolic Renewal. Akin suffered multiple cuts on her face in a 1987 car accident. Additionally, Akin's nose was "slashed and smashed sideways," she told reporters.

"The tip of my nose was actually touching my left cheek," she continued. "I was rushed to a hospital [for] extensive facial surgery."

After Akin's injuries had healed, scars remained on her nose and under her eyes.

Completely Removed Scars!

Akin had resigned herself to living with the scars permanently until she read an article about the glycolic product.

For the first seven days after receiving her supply of the cream, Akin says, she used it twice daily, as recommended by the company. She began using it three times a day after seven days, however, because the improvement to her face was so dramatic. She said her scars faded completely within thirty days.

Fountain Of Youth Found In Fish!

Wrinkles, as we stated earlier, are caused or enhanced by sun damage. Similarly—as hair and nails use many of the same nutrients as skin—many women with sun-damaged skin also have fragile nails and hair.

Imedeen is an oral restorative for UV damaged skin that has also proven effective in combating brittle hair and nails! It is produced by combining nutrients essential for healthy skin with extracts from various marine plants and animals. These deep sea nutrients include marine plant proteins and extracts from certain types of fish cartilage and the shells of shrimp and crab.

One protein extracted from marine organisms is NADG (N-acetyl-D-glucosamine). Studies have shown NADG to have a repairing effect on skin. NADG is commonly used by dermatologists for treating dermatitis and other skin rashes, and one form of it has been successfully used to create artificial skin for burn victims.

Imedeen Feeds Your Starving Skin The Nutrients It Craves!

Research conducted by Dr. R.L. Ruberg has shown that a cofactor in the production of many enzymes necessary for healing damaged skin is zinc gluconate, a special form of zinc. Skin healing can be retarded by even a minor zinc deficiency, Dr. Ruberg's studies have shown.

Our chapter on prostate disorders explained why the diets of approximately 90% of Americans are deficient in zinc. With this in mind, it's no wonder that skin damage can be reversed when zinc supplements are taken!

More Nutrients That Our Skin Loves!

Calcium is another mineral needed by our skin (as well as our bones, nails, hair, and other connective tissues) to maintain its healthiness. Our bodies convert organic silica to a form of calcium readily used by our skin and connective tissues. Silica dioxide is used in Imedeen because it is one of the richest sources of organic silica.

One vital protein for healthy skin is collagen. L-ascorbic acid is a rare variation of the nutrient ascorbic acid, which, when taken orally, stimulates the production of collagen. One of America's leading dermatologists, Dr. Sheldon Pinnell of the Dermatology Department of Medicine at Duke University Medical Center, published research on L-ascorbic acid's collagen stimulating effects in the *Yale Journal of Biology and Medicine*.

NADG, zinc gluconate, silica dioxide and L-ascorbic acid are the essential ingredients in Imedeen.

Research Published In International Journal!

The aforementioned Dr. Allen Lassus published his research on Imedeen in the *Journal of International Medical Research*. In this journal, Dr. Lassus reports: "...photodamaged skin shows a wide spectrum of structural changes. A conspicuous feature is a huge accumulation of tangled, thickened and strikingly abnormal elastic fibres. This condition, termed 'elastosis'...is accompanied by a great loss of collagen..."

Dr. Lassus conducted double-blind, placebo-controlled studies of Imedeen. The study group was divided into subgroups. One of these subgroups consisted of women with moderate to severe solar elastosis who were treated with 0.5 grams of Imedeen daily for ninety days. A similar group of women was treated with placebos.

Reduces Cellulite And Repairs Brittle Hair And Nails As Well As Sun-Damaged Skin!

There was a "statistically significant" difference in the non-placebo group, Dr. Lassus concludes, "...an improvement in wrinkles, mottles and dryness was observed. All patients with brittle hair and nails showed normalization. Both skin thickness and the elasticity index increased. Imedeen repaired clinical signs of solar elastosis, the effect of treatment usually starting after sixty days. No adverse effects were reported by the patients or observed by the investigators."

Additionally, several women in Dr. Lassus's study reported a reduction in cellulite, which is essentially a skin problem.

Dermatein: An Improved Version Of Imedeen!

The essential formula for Imedeen is now incorporated in a pill manufactured in the United States. This pill goes by the trade name Dermatein and is billed by its manufacturer, Gero Vita Laboratories, as a "significantly improved version of the original beauty from within a pill."

Gero Vita has added to its formula vitamin A, a nutrient important to the healthy metabolism of our outer layer of skin. Vitamin A also functions as an important anti-oxidant.

Another anti-oxidant addition to this newer formula is DL-alpha tocopheryl acetate, which stops free radicals. Research has shown that free radicals are the major cause of aging because they kill cells of the organs. As a major organ, our skin is most vulnerable to free radical attacks, which can cause age spots and deepen wrinkles.

Not A Cure, But An Ounce Of Prevention!

The "oral cosmetic" phycogene, also known as proanthocyandine or PAC, was originally used to treat skin and vein diseases. It was later found to prevent early facial wrinkles!

When Dr. Jacques Masquelier of Bordeaux University in France began his PAC studies, he researched the drug's effects on eczema, ulcerated varicose veins and related disorders. Later research prompted Dr. Masquelier to report in two medical journals that PAC, when taken soon enough, can prevent early facial wrinkles.

PAC Helps Bring Back Skin's Elasticity!

This is how PAC helps prevent wrinkles: Collagen is the underlying protein of our skin which maintains its texture and elasticity. PAC reacts with damaged collagen to bind its fibers and protect it from such harmful elements as free radicals and collagen-degrading enzymes. In so doing, PAC realigns the collagen fibers into a form that gives skin a smoother, more youthful appearance.

In addition to collagen's benefits on wrinkles and skin and vein conditions, the research of Dr. Stewart Brown, a gastroenterologist at the England's University of Nottingham, has shown that PAC helps to prevent stomach ulcers.

Skin Diseases: More Than Just A Nuisance!

Many of us find it difficult emotionally to deal with the cosmetic aspect of skin blemishes. As former Miss America Susan Akin put it, "My self-esteem and self-confidence really suffered [due to facial scars]. People stared at me, and I couldn't handle people feeling sorry for me."

Skin diseases, however, are often more difficult for people to endure than scars or the process of aging. In addition to any emotional trauma, sufferers of skin disorders must deal with annoyances ranging from itching to mild discomfort to severe pain.

New Hope For Shingles Sufferers!

Shingles (herpes-zoster) is one such painful skin disease. It affects nerves. Symptoms usually include pain and small skin blisters that form directly over the nerves involved. The nerves most commonly affected are those of the face, ribs, chest and spine.

Conventional treatments for shingles include pain killers, tranquilizers, steroids, and ultrasound and hot and cold packs. Less conventional treatments are acupuncture, chiropractic adjustments, biofeedback and bee propolis. A chiropractor can sometimes stop the disorder if it is diagnosed early enough. But unfortunately, while most remedies bring some relief to shingles symptoms, they don't treat its cause.

A study published recently in the *Journal of the American Academy of Dermatology*, however, documents the seemingly miraculous relief experienced by shingles sufferers who used the salve Zostrix. The active ingredient in Zostrix is the cayenne pepper extract capsaicin. Capsaicin has long been known to improve circulation and relieve intestinal gas when taken internally.

Twelve shingles patients at Case Western University participated in a capsaicin study conducted by Dr. David Bickers. The patients were instructed to apply a salve containing .025% capsaicin to their diseased skin five times daily the first week, followed by three times daily for an additional three weeks. At the end of four weeks 25% of the patients reported that their pain was completely gone! Another 50% gained substantial relief.

Echinacea!

Echinacea has been used by people throughout the world and the ages as a virtual cure-all for skin ailments. Several studies have been recorded that document *Echinacea's* benefits when either mixed in an ointment and used topically or when ingested orally.

An Ointment For All Sorts Of Skin Conditions!

A German study of 4,598 patients documented an *Echinacea* ointment's relief of an incredible array of skin conditions. The study reported an overall success rate of about 85% when the ointment was applied to skin areas affected with varicose leg ulcers, eczema (also known as dermatitis), wounds, abscesses, herpes simplex and foliculitis (inflammation of hair follicles).

"Generally the symptoms of pain, irritation, itching, etc, were gone within four days," Dr. David Williams reported. "In almost 90% of the cases involving wounds, burns, and herpes simplex the associated lesions disappeared within seven days. Significant improvement was seen in 83% of the eczema patients and 71% of those with leg ulcers."

A Natural Antibiotic!

A study cited in the journal *Planta Medica* documents *Echinacea's* usefulness for stimulation of the immune system's production of interferon. Interferon consists of one or more proteins formed when cells are exposed to viruses. It combats viral infection in the body. The study also concluded that *Echinacea* stimulates production in our bodies of T-lymphocytes (or T-cells) and other white blood cells. (Lymphocytes provide cellular immunity by acting against antigens such as bacterial toxins.)

Echinacea is an effective medicine for treating a wide array of skin conditions associated with toxicity, such as acne, skin eruptions and boils. This is because our lymphatic system will often become overworked when our bodies harbor infection and disease. *Echinacea* stimulates macrophage activity, which keeps our lymphatic system running at a healthy pace. Macrophages are large cells in our lymph nodes which act like battle submarines: they seek the enemy and the filter and destroy bacteria and other foreign particles circulating in our lymph fluid.

Beehive Cement Treats Skin Conditions!

What do acne, warts, burns, bedsores (decubitus ulcers) and herpes all have in common? They can all be treated—and benefited—by propolis.

Propolis is a brownish, resinous, waxy substance which is collected by bees from the buds of trees and used as beehive cement. It contains high concentrations of flavonoids, which are aromatic compounds that include many common pigments. Some of the flavonoids found in propolis are extremely potent antioxidants.

Russian Studies Document Propolis' Effects On Skin!

Propolis has incredible skin healing properties. Extensive studies on hundreds of patients in Russia have testified as to this beehive cement's antibiotic, bactericidal, anesthetic and regenerative qualities. One Russian study demonstrated that a 30% propolis ointment applied to severe skin conditions twice a day brought on better, faster healing than sulfur-based creams or the commonly prescribed antibiotic tetracycline!

In Russian hospitals during the 1960s, the most commonly used topical healing salve was an ointment made of 15% propolis in a vegetable fat base. The Russians also use it as a remedy for chronic inflammatory diseases and various kinds of ulcers. These include skin ulcerations to the lower legs, varicose ulcers, ulcerating bedsores, and ulcerations brought on by arteriosclerosis.

Further Research Reveals More Promising Benefits!

Bulgarian doctors have reported that propolis, when used to treat burns, demonstrated better, faster skin regeneration than most traditional treatments! Propolis ointment dressings have an added plus: They don't stick to burn wounds, making dressing changes simple, quick and, best of all, painless!

Bulgarian scientists are also reporting that a derivative of propolis has been very effective on enhancing the immune systems of laboratory animals.

At Poland's Silesian School of Medicine, studies have shown that yet another propolis derivative protects lab animals from gamma radiation.

Strong Antiviral Qualities!

Researchers at London's National Heart & Lung Institute have found that propolis combats the potentially fatal TB virus, (tubercle bacilli)!

When used topically, propolis can fight acne, warts and at least two herpes viruses: herpes zoster (shingles) and herpes simplex (which causes fever blisters and cold sores).

Propolis can potentially cause allergic reactions. Users should test just a small amount at first. Users should also be aware that topical application of the beehive cement will cause temporary inflammation to the treated area. As with all medications you should first consult a doctor—preferably one who is nutritionally oriented—before taking propolis.

Sources Of Other Substances
Listed In This Chapter:

Propolis can be obtained from beekeepers and many health food stores. It can also be purchased through two mail-order firm, C.C. Pollen Co., 3627 E. Indian School Rd., Ste. 209, Phoenix, AZ 85018-5126. Their toll free phone number is 1-800-875-0096.

Gero Vita GH3 Mature Skin Revitalizer and Dermatein are available by mail from Gero Vita International, Dept. Z101, 2255-B Queen Street East #820, Toronto, Ontario M4E 1G3, Canada, or call (800) 825-8482.

Skin Secrets Glycolic Renewal's name has been changed to "New Cell Therapy" and is available from L & H Vitamins. Call 1-800-221-1152. Vitamin A ointment is commonly called "retinol" cream which you may find at your local health food or vitamin store. L & H Vitamins also stocks it.

Imedeen tablets are produced by Ime-Enterprises of Switzerland. They are also available in the United States from Health Fest, 74 - 20th St., Brooklyn, N.Y. 11001.

Zostrix is produced by the GenDerm Corporation of Northbrook, Illinois, and is also available without prescription at many drugstores. *Echinacea* ointment (called pure Echinacea liquid extract) can be purchased at health food or vitamin stores.

12

New Scientific Wa
To Lose Weight An
Keep It Off!

I'm Too Fat, You're Too Fat!

At one time or another just about everybody has wanted to lose som
weight. Sometimes the reason for losing weight is personal, like lookin
good for the upcoming summer bathing suit season or next month's wed-
ding reception, or just being able to bend over and tie one's own shoes.
Sometimes the reason for weight-loss is medical: heart problems, high
blood pressure, diabetes.

Food, Food Everywhere!

But how we love to eat: pizza, hot fudge sundaes, fried chicken,
cheesecake, eggs Benedict, *duck à l'orange*, lasagne.

Of course, we have all heard that the only way we can lose weight
and keep it off is to start a strict exercise regimen and to change our diets
by cutting calories. And we all know that exercise requires a major time
and energy commitment while eating those boring, low calorie diet foods
which are no fun at all.

If only there was some pill or magic formula we could take to get the weight off!

Skipping Breakfast Does Not Work!

Remember how our mothers would always tell us that breakfast is the most important meal of the day? Well, many people ignore what mom said and try to cut back on the amount of calories they consume each day by skipping breakfast.

Guess what? Studies show that mom was right about breakfast! According to a study of dieters published in the *American Journal of Clinical Nutrition* by Vanderbilt University scientist Dr. David G. Schlundt, breakfast eaters lost more weight than breakfast skippers. The study noted that, contrary to the breakfast skippers' aim of cutting calories, the actual result was that passing up the morning meal induced hunger and encouraged high calorie snacking later.

Dr. Schlundt determined that "meal skipping may influence adherence to calorie controlled diet by encouraging overeating later in the day or by increasing between meal snacking on foods with poor nutrient density."

In other words, if you skip meals you will end up being so hungry that you'll eat a whole lot of fattening junk food.

We're Still In The Ice Age!

The human body has a fat producing trigger mechanism that seems to be left over from the Ice Age. As reported in the publication *Intelli-Scope,* in an article titled "Natural Fat-loss," humans developed the ability to store energy in the form of fat in order to survive 10,000 years ago. This ability came in handy since there were long periods of famine due to scarcity of food during winter periods. This stored body fat gave us the warmth and energy we needed to survive.

The fat producing survival mechanism is still part of our genetic makeup, and it is triggered when we skip meals.

"The bottom line," says noted author and life extension scientist Durk Pearson, "is that, if you want to get rid of body fat, caloric restriction—not eating when you're hungry—is the ultimate unnatural act. Your genes are telling you you're going to die if you do this, and in fact, when people lose weight too fast with any technique, the master control center in their brain will actually alter their metabolism to make it very difficult to lose further fat, because that fat is their Ice Age life insurance policy."

Eating Is Important To Weight Reduction!

Dr. Schlundt points out that eating breakfast, in addition to minimizing impulsive snacking, seems to provide many benefits that include reducing a person's daily intake of fat, maintaining a more constant blood sugar level and improving strength and endurance.

Eating breakfast, Dr. Schlundt concludes in his weight loss study, "may be an important part of a weight reduction program." Further, he recommends that "individuals attempting a weight loss program include a breakfast that is low in fat and high in carbohydrates as part of their weight loss regimen," since eating the morning meal discourages snacking in general and encourages healthier snacks when snacking does occur.

The Failure Of Cutting Calories!

Cutting back on our caloric intake in order to lose weight just does not do the job. "People who try to lose weight by drastically cutting calories often fail," states Dr. Hans Kugler, vice president of the National Health Federation.

And, as reported in *Intelli-Scope*, about 95% of those people who lose weight using the calorie deprivation method gain all of those lost pounds back within a year.

What Do We Do Now?

Now we know that if we torture ourselves by avoiding meals and cutting calories, our chances at permanent weight loss are poor. It is beginning to seem hopeless, so what can we do to lose weight?

One of the more conventional solutions to the weight loss dilemma is thyroid supplements, which speed up the activity of the thyroid gland and burn off weight.

Unfortunately, thyroid medication must be administered under a doctor's care and is generally given only to obese people with underactive thyroids.

FDA Does Not Like Non-Prescription Diet Drugs!

For the rest of us, we need to fall back on less conventional supplements if we want to lose weight. Happily, there are many highly successful weight loss formulas and supplements available both through prescription and over-the-counter.

These pills, powders and herbal teas that can help us lose weight are available despite the federal government's efforts to limit our access to them. As reported by *The New York Times*, the Food and Drug Administration (FDA) has banned 111 ingredients used in non-prescription diet drugs because, the FDA contends, these ingredients do not work.

Take A Supplement And Eat Less!

Dietary weight loss supplements fall into two basic categories: appetite suppressants and fat burners.

DL-phenylalanine (DLPA) is a natural appetite suppressant. It is an essential amino acid (which means that DLPA cannot be made by the body but has to be supplied from outside sources) used clinically to treat depression and chronic pain.

From our standpoint, the good thing about DLPA is that it causes the brain to release cholecystokinin (CCK), a hormone that inhibits appetite. CCK has a gradual effect that makes eating seem less important, rather than causing outright rejection of food. The hormone tends to make person feel full on much smaller amounts of food than they would normally need. DLPA requires no prescription and is available from those sources that supply your everyday vitamin and mineral supplements, such as health food stores and vitamin and nutrition centers.

Researchers Find A Way
To Kill The Craving For Fat!

In the continuing search by scientists to come up with a magic formula that will keep us all from eating too much, researchers have come across a brain chemical called galanin. Galanin, it seems, increases the desire to eat fat. The researchers have also come up with an experimental drug that blocks the effects of galanin, killing the craving for fat.

"Galanin," says Dr. Sarah Leibowitz of Rockefeller University in New York City, "is the only brain chemical found that directly correlates with fat intake." Its discovery, she states, has important implications for medical problems that revolve around obesity and eating disorders. The finding of and testing for galanin, according to Dr. Leibowitz, may help doctors determine which children will be most susceptible to high fat diets.

Dr. Leibowitz also found a substance that blocks the effects of galanin. Testing has been done and that magic pill to suppress our fat craving may be just a few years away.

The Magic Pill!

Or is that magic pill here already? Fitting into the fat burning category of dietary supplements is Orlistat (chemical name: tetrahydrolipstatin), which was developed by New Jersey-based Hoffman-La Roche. Essentially, the chemical keeps fat from getting into the bloodstream.

A recent test of dieters who took Orlistat showed them losing twice as much weight as those dieters in the control group.

Does this mean that if we took Orlistat, we could eat as much fat as we wanted? The answer is no, says Dr. Jonathan Hauptman, director of therapeutic research at Hoffman-La Roche. No matter how much of the chemical we take it will only prevent 90% of the fat we eat from being digested.

Nevertheless, even with its limitations, Orlistat shows great promise as a weight loss aid. The drug does need FDA approval, however, and may not be on the market for several years.

MCT Reduces Fat!

While Orlistat may not be available yet, there are other fat burners on the market. Studies have found that medium-chain triglycerides (MCTs), a non-prescription product, reduce fat deposits by converting them into energy. MCTs change the pattern of fat metabolism so that more fat is used for energy and much less fat stored.

"MCTs," says nutritionist Dr. Allan Geliebter, "may have potential for dietary prevention of human obesity." A study of animals given MCT showed that these animals gained less weight and had a lower fat content than the group that was not fed MCT. The study was conducted at Harvard Medical School's Nutrition/Metabolism Laboratory and headed by Dr. Pei-Ra Ling, a visiting researcher from Peking Union Medical College.

"MCT reduces the fat deposition without reducing the whole body protein content," concluded Dr. Ling.

More Fat Burners!

L-carnitine, an amino acid that is essential for fat metabolism, can be used in conjunction with MCT. Studies show that l-carnitine significantly lowers blood fat levels and is very powerful when taken in combination with MCT.

Since we are not able to convert all of the food we eat into energy right away, and the excess gets stored as fat. Coenzyme Q1O is another supplement that helps us in this regard because it enhances energy production, thereby reducing fat storage.

Reduce Fat And Increase Muscle!

Chromium picolinate is a mineral that is more than just an effective weight management tool. Studies show that it reduces body fat while building lean muscle.

In a Louisiana State University study, women taking chromium picolinate gained 80% more lean muscle and had significantly greater increases in measurement of chests, arms and thighs than women taking a placebo.

In addition, chromium picolinate provides the added advantages of lowering cholesterol and blood sugar levels.

Thermogenesis: The Body's Natural Furnace!

Our bodies have two kinds of fat cells: white fat cells (where energy is stored) and brown fat cells that burn the white cells, releasing their energy. The fat burning process is called thermogenesis, and anything that can increase this natural process makes it possible for us to lose weight without dieting.

The basis for all thermogenic enhancers is the Ephedra herb, an herb that has been used for centuries in the Orient, often in the form of MA Haung tea, for relief of asthma, nasal congestion and gastric cramps.

Clinical studies with obese individuals showed that the Ephedra's effects are enhanced by extended use. Without either dieting or exercising subjects lost an average of a pound a week for twelve weeks.

Ephedra!

Dr. Kugler of the National Health Federation recommends Vita Trim, a natural thermogenic dietary supplement that contains *Ephedra sinica* and *Camellia sinsensis*. The two herbs, he says, suppress appetite as well as increase the rate at which the body burns fat.

Vitamin Research Products (VRP) provides several weight management formulas that contain *Ephedra*. Thermo 'T' is an instant herbal tea, while Thermogenic Enhancer combines *Ephedra*, niacin and caffeine in a capsule. Another VRP product is ThermaLoss, which blends *Ephedra*, l-carnitine and taurine, an antioxidant.

Dymetadrine 25 is an over-the-counter drug that is used to treat bronchial spasms, but it is actually pure natural ephedrine, the drug derived from Ephedra.

A Hormone That Helps!

One of the more amazing substances that may eventually become a potent weapon in the battle against the bulge is dehydroepiandrosterone (DHEA), a hormone that is produced by the adrenal glands of mammals that can also be derived from the Mexican yam.

According to Dr. Arthur Schwartz, a Temple University microbiologist, DHEA enhances the body's thermogenic process, thereby transforming food into energy and preventing fat from accumulating.

A study at Temple University's School of Medicine found that DHEA caused weight loss without a change in appetite. Weight loss occurred because calories were converted to heat rather than to fat.

Dr. Terence T. Yen, a biochemist at Eli Lilly, conducted a study that showed significant weight loss in obese mice who were fed DHEA.

Although our bodies produce DHEA naturally, at about age 25 production begins to decline, necessitating our taking DHEA supplementation.

Reduced Body Fat By One Third!

Studies of mice indicate that in addition to the weight loss benefit there are other reasons to take DHEA. The hormone increased life expectancy and reduced the risk of developing several forms of cancer.

Dr. Schwartz reported that DHEA reduced body fat by one third, prevented atherosclerosis and mitigated diabetes. He is working on a synthetic version of the hormone.

Currently, DHEA is hard to get in the United States, as its use is discouraged by the FDA.

Sources Of Substances Mentioned
In This Chapter:

Thyroid supplements are available with a doctor's prescription.

Dl-phenylalanine can be obtained from some health food and vitamin stores and from Vitamin Research Products (VRP), 3579 Hwy. 50 East, Carson City, NV 89701, (800) 877-2447.

L-carnitine and coenzyme Q10 can be purchased at vitamin and health food stores and can be ordered from VRP.

MCT (medium-chain triglycerides) can be purchased some vitamin and health food stores. MCT Oil is also available from Gero Vita International, Dept. Z101, 2255-B Queen Street East #820, Toronto, Ontario M4E 1G3, Canada, or call (800) 825-8482.

Chromium picolinate is available from VRP, health food and vitamin stores.

Vita Trim can be purchased from Gero Vita International.

Thermo T, Thermogenic Enhancer, ThermaLoss can be ordered from VRP.

DHEA may be obtained from Belmar Pharmacy, 8015 W. Alameda Ave., Suite 100, Lakewood, CO, (880) 525-9473; and College Pharmacy, 833 N. Tejon St., Colorado Springs, CO, (800) 748-2263.

Vita Potencia, made by Gero Vita International, contains naturally-occuring DHEA from Mexican wild yam.

13

New Remedies For Arthritis And Rheumatism!

More than 32 million individuals, approximately 14% of the nation's population, suffer from one form or another of arthritis—an inflammatory joint affliction. Sixteen million have been diagnosed with osteoarthritis, a disease of joint cartilage with associated secondary changes in the underlying bone. Some 6.5 million others are diagnosed with rheumatoid arthritis, also known as rheumatism.

Osteoarthritis commonly affects the hip, knee and thumb joints. It is most prevalent in those past middle life and results from degeneration of the protective cartilage surrounding the joint through years of use or injury. Eventually the rough, unprotected surfaces of bone painfully rub against each other.

Rheumatoid arthritis, according to the American Rheumatism Foundation, is most common in the hips, elbow, shoulders, fingers, and wrists, and found less often in the knees, sacrum, heels and toes. This type of arthritis destroys the cartilage and tissues in and around the joints. Scar tissue replaces the destroyed tissue with the space between the joints fusing together in the later stages of the disease.

Both types of arthritis can cause extreme pain resulting from the inflammation of the affected joints.

The Immune Connection!

Rheumatoid arthritis has been related to a dysfunctional immune system. The body's antibodies are in some way deficient and unable to distinguish between invading organisms and healthy cells and thus attack both. Immune complexes are typically present in the joint fluid and serum.

The disease is systemic and initially appears with general immune-related symptoms such as fatigue, weakness, poor appetite, low-grade fever and anemia. Unlike osteoarthritis, which generally is found among older people or former athletes, rheumatoid arthritis tends to strike individuals in their thirties and forties and is far more common among women than men. Because it is a systemic condition, rheumatoid arthritis can progress from one joint to many others.

Conventional Treatment Is Expensive!

The Arthritis Foundation estimates that Americans spend more than $5 billion a year to ease the pain of their arthritis.

The physician's conventional approach to arthritis is the prescription of nonsteroidal anti-inflammatory drugs (NSAIDs), which are very costly and are no more effective than inexpensive over-the-counter medications.

In a recent study by Dr. Kenneth D. Brandt at the Indiana University School of Medicine, reported in the *New England Journal of Medicine*, it was shown that osteoarthritic patients who took over-the-counter medications did just as well as those who took the expensive, prescribed NSAIDs.

And Worse Yet, It's Dangerous!

NSAIDs, when used on a chronic basis, can be extremely dangerous. Each year 25,000 people suffer from gastrointestinal tract bleeding as a direct result of ingesting prescribed NSAIDs.

The very drugs that are being prescribed for arthritis can in actuality accelerate cartilage destruction. In a recent Norway study of osteoarthritic patients taking Indocin, a strong NSAID, it was found that those taking the Indocin had far more rapid destruction of the hip than the group that was not taking Indocin or any other NSAID.

In a recently published report in the *Journal of the American Medical Association*, physicians based in New York and Boston reported on the severe liver damage caused by Voltaren, one of the nation's most frequently prescribed NSAIDs for arthritis. Patients developed hepatitis within four to six weeks of taking the medication, and one died from liver damage several weeks after starting on the drug.

Beware Of Nonprescription Remedies!

Even over-the-counter anti-inflammatories and analgesics (pain relievers) such as Anacin, Bufferin, Bayer (containing aspirin); Advil, Motrin, Nuprin (containing ibuprofen); and Tylenol, Datril, Pandol (containing acetaminophen) can have disastrous side effects.

The mechanism of action of aspirin, ibuprofen and acetaminophen is actually the same as the prescription NSAIDs—they block the action of prostaglandins, chemical messengers involved in the inflammatory process.

They Cause Ulcers!

Prostaglandins, however, have other, more useful functions in the body—one being to maintain the protective mucosal lining of the stomach. Twenty percent of the 20 million Americans who take large doses of these nonprescription NSAIDs for arthritis develop serious gastric ulcers. Each year 10,000 of these individuals die from hemorrhages.

Kidney failure is another alarming potential side effect of NSAIDs, particularly in individuals whose blood flow is diminished by age or other medications.

Nutritional Depletion!

If you have arthritis, you are probably nutritionally depleted as well. Dr. George Moore, head of six arthritis clinics in Southern California and a recognized arthritis expert, notes that the majority of the arthritic patients seen at his clinics are malnourished, exhibiting deficiencies in zinc, B vitamins, and vitamin C. Dr. Robert Bingham reports in the *Journal of the Academey of Rheumatoid Diseases* that nutritional supplements correct 80% to 90% of all arthritis cases.

Amazing Amino Acid
Protects Endorphins!

DL-Phenylalanine (DLPA), a natural amino acid found in many of the foods you eat, is a powerful, nonaddictive analgesic. Dr. Earl L. Mindell, author of *The Vitamin Bible*, notes that DLPA is as or more effective in relieving pain as morphine or other opiates.

When you are injured or experiencing disease, your body naturally produces morphine-like chemicals called endorphins. At the same time, however, certain enzymes are programmed to destroy the endorphins. DLPA works by inhibiting the enzymes, thus allowing the endorphins to continue their pain relief activities.

A study by Dr. Reuben Balagot, a University of Chicago anesthesiologist, found that a single dose of DLPA increased the activity of a small brain endorphin believed to be involved in the analgesic response. This is highly significant because people with arthritis have a lower level of endorphins than do those without the disease.

The first clinical research on DLPA was presented at the Second World Congress on Pain by Dr. Seymour Ehrenpreis of the University of Chicago Medical School and subsequently published in *Advances in Pain Research and Therapy*. Good to excellent pain relief with no adverse effects was noted in every patient, each of whom had been unresponsive to conventional pain treatment.

170

A follow-up study in the *Journal of Endogenous and Exogenous Opiate Agonists and Antagonists* found that the most profound pain relief experienced was in a subset of osteoarthritic patients. A double blind study conducted at the Royal Infirmary in England showed similar DLPA pain relief results.

DLPA Is Synergistic And Long-Lasting!

One of the unique qualities of DLPA is that it works synergistically with any other existing therapy—NSAIDs, acupuncture, physical therapy, chiropractic—often with results more beneficial than those achieved by any single therapy. You don't need to change what you are currently doing; simply add DLPA to your treatment program.

Once the pain relief effects of DLPA are established, the body can remain pain free without the continual ingestion of the amino acid. Most studies of chronic pain patients using DLPA have shown that patients need only take DLPA two weeks out of the month.

Amino Acid Stimulates Bone Growth And Enhances Immunity!

Another amino acid, l-arginine, helps arthritis sufferers by stimulating the growth of new bone and tendon cells. It appears that ingestion of arginine increases human growth hormone (HGH), which in turn accelerates the formation of new bone and tendon.

When healthy males were given a single oral dose of arginine, reported Dr. A. Isidori in *Current Medical Research and Opinion*, a definite increase in HGH was noted in all subjects, often occurring as rapidly as within 30 minutes of the intake of the amino acid.

Arginine research has also shown it to be an immunoenhancer, stimulating the thymus gland and boosting lymphocyte (white blood cell) production in the gland. Several studies by Dr. A. Barbul published in the *Journal of Parenteral and Enteral Nutrition, Surgery and Surgical Forum* have documented this vital role.

Two Important B Vitamins!

As Dr. Moore and other physicians have noted, arthritis patients typically are deficient in B vitamins. Research has shown that two specific B vitamins—pantothenic acid (part of the B-complex) and niacin (B_3)—are helpful in treating arthritis.

Research conducted by Dr. Barton-Wright and published in *Lancet* revealed that the whole blood pantothenic acid level of individuals with rheumatoid arthritis was significantly lower than those without the disease. Moreover, the lower the level of the vitamin, the more severe were the symptoms.

A double blind study of rheumatoid arthritis patients by the General Practitioner Research Group reported in *Practitioner* that the group given pantothenic acid showed a significant reduction in duration of morning stiffness, severity of pain and degree of disability, in comparison to the control group which experienced no significant improvements.

Dr. William Kaufman has published several reports regarding the effectiveness of niacin in the relief of arthritis symptoms, while Nobel laureate Dr. Linus Pauling has noted the effectiveness of niacin in treating arthritis when it is combined with vitamin C.

Vitamin C Achieves Results!

The levels of vitamin C were found to be significantly decreased in the leucocytes and plasma of rheumatoid arthritis patients in a study reported by Dr. Mullen in *Proceedings of Nutritional Science*. This finding, the study proposed, was probably due to increased degradation and excretion of vitamin C in response to inflammation.

Dr. Linus Pauling, in his book *How to Live Longer and Feel Better*, explains that in diseases like rheumatoid arthritis, substances are released into the blood that interfere with phagocyte mobility. Vitamin C supplements have been found by many investigators to improve the activity of these immune cells.

One of the most dramatic and well-known examples of the power of vitamin C therapy was the case of Norman Cousins, the former editor of the *Saturday Review* and later a prominent medical lecturer, researcher and author of *Anatomy Of An Illness*, *The Healing Heart* and *Head First*.

Cousins successfully overcame a particularly crippling form of arthritis—ankylosing spondylitis—through a combination of high dosage vitamin C infusions and laughter. He checked himself out of the hospital and into a hotel room, where he received high dosage vitamin C intravenously and watched comedy videos. He recounts this experience in *Anatomy Of An Illness*.

Zinc Zings Arthritis!

The mineral zinc is essential for the normal functioning of joints. It is no surprise then that lower levels of serum zinc are found in rheumatoid arthritics than in nonafflicted individuals. A study by Dr. W. Niedermeier in the *Journal of Chronic Diseases* and a later study by Dr. S. P. Pandey in the *Indian Journal of Medical* Research validate this finding.

A double blind study conducted by Dr. P.A. Simkin and published in *Lancet* reported significant initial reductions in morning stiffness and joint swelling. The benefits to the treatment group, which was given zinc sulfate, continued, which was not the case with the control group.

Another double blind study by Dr. O.J. Clemmensen of patients with psoriatic arthritis (inflammatory arthritis coupled with the skin disease psoriasis), published in the *British Journal of Dermatology*, revealed similar relief of rheumatoid symptoms with zinc supplementation.

Iron-Poor Blood!

Anemia may be one of the symptoms of reheumatoid arthritis. Dr. W. Niedermeir reported in the *Journal of Chronic Disease* that patients with rheumatoid arthritis had significantly reduced levels of iron in their blood serum compared to those without the disease.

A recent study in the *Scandinavian Journal of Rheumatology* by Dr. M. Hansen notes the positive results achieved in patients with rheumatoid arthritis who received iron supplements.

Equisetum arvense, commonly known as horsetail, is an excellent natural source of silica, a trace mineral found in highest concentrations in bone, connective tissue, fingernails, and skin. Horsetail is also rich in calcium and several other minerals needed to rebuild injured tissue and is thus helpful in the healing of arthritis.

Nontoxic Glucosamine Builds Connective Tissue!

Glucosamine is found in high concentrations in between joints, where it acts to stimulate the production of connective tissue—the primary component of cartilage. Supplemental glucosamine sulfate not only has been shown to be an effective analgesic, but it has the potential for actually repairing arthritic joints by stimulating the growth of new cartilage.

As was mentioned previously, NSAIDs are toxic drugs with side effects that may cause extreme damage to the gastrointestinal tract, the liver and the kidneys. Glucosamine has no toxicity and is effective in treating arthritis.

It has been shown in a Portuguese double blind study by Dr. Antonio Lopez Vaz that glucosamine provided significant pain relief in those receiving the supplement, compared to the control group that took the NSAID ibuprofen.

Other studies in Italy have found glucosamine not only effective in relieving inflammation response, but concluded that because of its nontoxic nature, glucosamine was 10 to 30 times better for long term therapy than NSAIDs.

Pineapple That Heals!

Bromelain, found in pineapple, is a digestive enzyme that breaks down protein. It also has anti-inflammatory properties that have been scientifically shown to be effective in the treatment of rheumatoid arthritis.

In a study by Dr. A. Cohen, reported in the *Pennsylvania Medical Journal*, over 70% of the participants, some of whom had both rheumatoid and osteoarthritis, experienced excellent to good results of decreased pain and joint swelling and increased mobility.

Hot Pepper Cools Arthritis!

Red cayenne pepper contains five different capsaicins—the ingredient that makes it hot—and that also makes it a pain reliever for arthritis.

Capsaicin blocks substance P, a neuropeptide produced by the nerves that carry pain sensation. This blocking activity makes capsaicin a long-lasting anesthetic. In double blind studies skin ointments containing capsaicin have been shown to significantly relieve the pain of arthritis.

Copper Folk Remedy Proven Scientifically!

Despite the skepticism of the medical community, the folk remedy of wearing a copper bracelet to combat arthritis has persisted. Now medical researchers have actually investigated this practice.

In a double blind study by Dr. Walker, published in *Agents and Actions*, it was found that the osteoarthritic participants who wore copper bracelets worsened after discontinuing their use, whereas those wearing placebo bracelets exhibited no change in their symptoms. With evidence suggesting that the copper was absorbed through the skin, researchers began to look a little closer at this folk remedy.

A number of studies by Dr. Niedermier published in the *Annals of Rheumatic Disease and the Journal of Chronic Disease* have shown that victims of rheumatoid arthritis have increased blood levels of copper in comparison to those without the disease.

Originally, researchers thought that increased levels of copper meant that it was the cause of the disease. Now it is known that the trace mineral copper is a protector, and that the higher blood levels are indicative of the body's attempt to fight inflammatory disease.

Several studies have shown that copper salicylate (copper complexed with aspirin) is more effective for arthritic pain relief than aspirin or copper taken individually. One study of 1,140 patients given short-term intravenous copper salicylate found that 89% experienced remission of fever, decreased swelling and increased joint mobility for an average of over three years.

Superoxide Dimutase Partners With Copper!

Superoxide dimutase (SOD) is one of the body's natural antioxidants that scavenge free radicals—those highly charged molecules that have been shown to accelerate the aging process.

When the enzyme SOD is complexed with copper into copper superoxide dismutase it has both antioxidant and anti-inflammatory properties. Injections of copper-zinc SOD directly into arthritic joints have been shown to be effective in several studies: by Dr. K. M. Goebel reported in *Lancet*, by Dr. K. B. Menander-Huber reported in the *European Journal of Rheumatologic Inflammation*, and by Dr. M. Walraven published in *Current Therapy Research*. These trials were conducted on patients with osteoarthritis and rheumatoid arthritis.

More Than A Blooming Cactus!

Yucca, also known as Spanish bayonet, is a cactus that flourishes in the Southwestern desert. It has traditionally been used by the desert natives as both food and medicine.

Evidence is now available that yucca is particularly useful in the relief of arthritis. A double blind study by Dr. R. Bingham of the National Arthritis Medical Clinic in California's Desert Hot Springs, reported in a *Journal of Applied Nutrition*, found that 61% of those who received the yucca extract experienced less pain, swelling and stiffness compared to 23% of those individuals receiving the placebo.

Another Healing Cactus!

Aloe vera, a yucca-like plant, has been used for a variety of curative powers for centuries. *Aloe vera* contains more than 200 nutritional substances including salicylates, which have both anti-inflammatory and analgesic properties. An enzyme in *Aloe vera* has been found to inhibit bradykinin—a producer of pain in inflamed tissue.

Well-designed studies on animals have shown *Aloe vera* effective in inhibiting pain, blocking inflammation and restoring bone growth—in essence, both healing and arresting arthritis.

Fish Oils Also Help Arthritis!

Much has been learned in recent years about the beneficial cardio-vascular effects of fish oils. Now researchers are demonstrating that fish oils are also effective agents for relieving arthritis.

A recent double blind study in *Lancet* by Dr. J. M. Kremer described how the rheumatoid arthritis participants given fish oil supplements showed no further progression of the disease, while those receiving the placebos continued to worsen. A follow-up study by the same physician in *Annals of Internal Medicine* demonstrated similar results.

Shark Attacks Arthritis!

Sharks have supercharged immune systems which produce antibodies against viruses, bacteria and even toxic chemicals. Extracts of shark cartilage have anti-inflammatory properties helpful in treating arthritis.

A double blind, five year study by Dr. V. Rejholec of Czechoslovakia's Charles University compared a group of osteoarthritic patients who took a placebo with the addition of NSAIDs during flare-ups with those given shark cartilage. The findings, reported in *Seminars in Arthritis and Rheumatism*, revealed that those using the cartilage had a 85% decrease in pain scores compared to a 5% decrease in the placebo group. Also, the joint degeneration in the group using shark cartilage was only 37% of that of the control group.

Dr. Jose Orcasita notes the beneficial effects of shark cartilage in his clinical study of osteoarthritic patients at the University of Miami School of Medicine. All patients, with one exception, experienced a decrease in pain of four to five points on a ten point pain scale, increased mobility and joint inflammation reduction.

Joint cartilage is composed mainly of water, collagen and glycosaminoglycan. The primary component of glycosaminoglycan is chondroitin sulfate, which a study in *Clinical Experiments in Rheumatology* has shown to be lower in individuals with arthritis than in those free of the disease. Numerous European studies have shown that oral dosages of this cartilage component can help repair damaged cartilage, and that it may be more readily absorbed in the digestive system than whole cartilage.

Supplement Sources!

The supplements mentioned in the foregoing are available from health food or vitamin stores: vitamin C, niacin (vitamin B3), pantothenic acid, zinc, iron, horsetail, l-arginine, Dl-phenylalanine, bromelain, capsaicin (cayenne), *Aloe vera* and fish oils,

A combination of many of these are included in ARTHRIL (containing Dl-Phenylalanine, l-arginine, horsetail, niacin, pantothenic acid, vitamin C, iron and zinc) available from Gero Vita International, Dept. Z101, 2255-B Queen Street East #820, Toronto, Ontario M4E 1G3, Canada, or call (800) 825-8482.

Although *Aloe vera* is usually available in health food and vitamin stores, many of the products are diluted with water. Other sources for the concentrate are:

Lametco
Castle Rock, CO
(800) 933-2565

Coats Aloe International
Dallas, TX
(800) 486-ALOE

R Pur-Aloe International
Northglenn, CO
(800) 888-2563

Aloe Complete
Vista, CA
(619) 279-0727

If you can't find cayenne capsules locally, they may be ordered from:

Heart Foods
1 (800) CAYENNE

An inexpensive form of capsaicin (cayenne) ointment called Satogesic Hot Gel is available at Walgreens and other pharmacies. If you can't find it in your area, contact:

Sato Pharmaceutical
(310) 793-0509

If unavailable locally, bromelain in either powdered form (Vitamin Research Products, Mountain View, CA) or capsules (Thompson) may be obtained at a discount from:

The Vitamin Shoppe
4700 Westside Avenue
North Bergen, NJ 07047
(800) 223-1216

Shark cartilage is available from:

Wholesale Nutrition
POB 3345
Saratoga, CA 95050-9942
(800) 325-2664

Gero Vita Laboratories
1350 Flamingo Road, Dept. Z100,
Las Vegas, NV 89119
(800) 825-8482.

Chondroitin sulfate products manufactured by Biotics Research Corporation (Houston, TX) and Cardiovascular Research (Concord, CA) may be purchased at a discount from:

The Vitamin Shoppe
4700 Westside Avenue
North Bergen, NJ 07047
(800) 223-1216

Yucca, glucosamine and copper salicylate may be available in health food and vitamin stores. If you don't find these supplements on the shelf, ask your local merchant to order them for you.

As superoxide dimutase (SOD) is only effective by injection, you will need to locate a nutritionally oriented physician who administers this treatment.

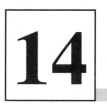

The Natural Way To Better Vision

Our eyes are our windows to the world. Yet nearly 143 million Americans suffer from vision problems that affect their view of the world. Unfortunately, many of these individuals are unaware of the array of natural substances that can help them maintain healthy eyes and good vision.

Numerous medical research studies confirm what many have believed for a long time: nutrients are effective in treating a wide variety of eye difficulties ranging from fatigue, to night blindness to cataracts. The scientific community is just now recognizing that many natural substances have legitimate medicinal applications for treating eye problems.

Bilberry Jam!

For hundreds of years, the bilberry plant (*Vaccinium myrtillus*), which grows wild in Northern Europe and Asia, has been used to make fresh jam. But it wasn't until World War II that the jam was discovered to have medicinal purposes. British Royal Air Force pilots found that when they ate bilberry jam before flying a mission, their night vision and visual acuity improved.

Since World War II, doctors and scientists all over the world have demonstrated the effectiveness of the bilberry fruit for treating a variety of visual problems. More than 50 scientific studies have been published confirming the value of the bilberry.

Not Just For Pilots!

Anyone who suffers from eye strain or scratchy, blurry, fatigued eyes can benefit from the healing effects of the bilberry plant. In Europe, bilberry anthocyanosides are the main ingredient in many over-the-counter treatments for eye problems. The substance has long been accepted as a remedy for maintaining healthy eyes and good vision.

The extract can help soothe tired eyes, which are problematic for many of those who read a lot, work at computers for long periods of time, drive long distances at night, or have difficulty adjusting to dim or bright light. There are boundless possible applications for the bilberry extract.

Relief From Eye Strain And Night Blindness!

The modern theory of vision is that how well you see and the ability of your eyes to adapt in dim light, are directly related to the amount of rhodopsin (visual purple) in the retinal rod of your eyes.

Dr. J.P. Baillart reported in a medical research journal, *Le Medicine de Reserve*, that your store of rhodopsin is depleted when you strain your eyes or when your eyes have to adjust to the dark.

As you age, your supply of rhodopsin also steadily decreases, resulting in poor vision. Anthocyanoside, the active ingredient in the bilberry fruit, has been found to actually stimulate the production of rhodopsin in the eye. In experiments with animals published in *C.R. Soc. Biology*, Dr. R. Alfieri determined that the bilberry extract accelerated the replenishment of rhodopsin and increased the speed of which the eye adapts to dark.

Improvement In Only Ten Days!

Dr. M. Ala El Din Barradah at the Ophthalmology Department of the University of Cairo substantiated the earlier findings of these scientists. Dr. Ala El Din Barradah's findings signify that bilberry extract could stop the development of nearsightedness and even reduce severe nearsightedness. According to a published report in the *Bulletin of the Ophthalmological Society of Egypt*, in only ten days, anthocyanoside improved visual acuity and night blindness in 100% of the severely nearsighted patients studied.

Other scientific studies have yielded similar results. A team of French scientists headed by Dr. G.E. Jayle found that in humans, bilberry extract improved visual acuity and improved vision during prolonged exposure to light. The study also concluded that subjects also experienced some improvement of vision in low light.

In addition, bilberry provides relief for tired eyes, according to Dr. E. Gil Del Rio in a study published in a French ophthalmological journal, *Gaz Med De France*.

Effective In Preventing Eye Disease And Improving Retinal Functioning

In a series of scientific studies published in *C.R. Soc. Biology* and *Biochemical Pharmacology*, Dr. C. Cluzel reported that the bilberry extract improved retinal functioning. As stated in the book *Guaranteed Potency Herbs: Next Generation Herbal Medicine*, "Bilberry anthocyanosides have a favorable affect on the operation of crucial enzymes in the retinal cellular metabolism and function..."

This amazing extract also tested positively for preventing the eye diseases associated with hypertension and diabetic-induced glaucoma, according to a study by Dr. B. Bever documented in the *Journal of Crude Drug Research*.

The results of clinical research reported by Dr. G. Zavarisse in a medical journal indicates that the bilberry ingredient also reduces sensitivity to light or day blindness. In addition, Dr. Zavarisse noted that no side effects to the bilberry treatment were experienced.

Relief Without Side Effects!

When taken orally, bilberry extract is completely non-toxic. Several other scientific trials uncovered corroborating evidence that the anthocyanocides provides relief for eye conditions without side effects, and that the effect of the herb gradually wears off over time. For medicinal substances, these are generally believed to be favorable attributes. Besides the obvious, this eliminates the need for extensive and costly experiments on the long-term effects of the substance on the body.

Link Found Between
Aspirin And Blindness!

The New England Journal of Medicine reported startling evidence of a corrclation between heavy aspirin consumption and macular degeneration (breaks in the blood vessels of the retina that can eventually lead to blindness).

Research indicates that bilberry and other nutrients, such as vitamin C, selenium, and zinc, can reduce clotting as well as aspirin can, without the risk of hemorrhaging that can lead to a loss of vision. Bilberry is one of the few treatments found effective in fighting this degenerative disease.

More Effective
Than Other Flavonoids!

Adding to the value of the bilberry, Dr. G. Demure published the results of a study in the European medical journal, *Medicine Clermont*, which demonstrated that the bilberry is more productive than other flavonoids (collectively known as vitamin P) in fighting the breakdown of the capillary walls.

The bilberry extract has also proven more effective than vitamin P in stimulating the production of rhodopsin (necessary for good vision), according to a study published by Dr. H. Pourrat in the journal, *Chim. Therapy.*

Because of their effect on decreasing the permeability of blood vessels, bilberries have also proven beneficial in treating other blood disorders. Health problems, such as ulcers and hypertension are also improved by bilberry treatment.

Dosage!

Proper dosage is dependent on the individual and the severity of the eye problem. For treating most eye conditions, two to four 25 mg capsules per day is recommended. For temporary or mild eyestrain, one day of treatment should provide appropriate relief. Higher doses have not been found to produce any negative side effects.

However, bilberry alone is not the answer. Studies indicate that there are other nutrients which are also essential for preventing visual disorders and maintaining healthy eyes.

Nutritional Supplements Provide Protection Against Cataracts!

It is estimated that 50 million people worldwide suffer from cataracts. A cataract is buildup of protein on the lens of the eye resulting in blurred vision and sometimes blindness. According to a study by the World Health Association, cataracts cause half the blindness in the world.

Most young people do not develop cataracts because normal eye functioning allows them to successfully clear the excess protein. However, exposure to the sun and dangerous ultraviolet rays can cause protein to build up on the eye and form cataracts over time.

New scientific evidence indicates that antioxidant nutrients, such as carotene, vitamin C and vitamin E, can protect eyes against the damage caused by ultraviolet light. According to Dr. H. Gerster in a report published in a Swiss medical journal, *Ernahrungswissenschaft*, "Different animal species have demonstrated a significant protective effect of vitamins C and E against light-induced cataract. Sugar and steroid cataracts were prevented as well. Epidemiological evidence in humans suggests that persons with comparatively higher intakes or blood concentrations of antioxidant vitamins are at a reduced risk of cataract development."

Vitamin C and E!

Nobel Prize winner Dr. Linus Pauling states in his book *How to Live Longer & Feel Better*, that "the importance of ascorbate (vitamin C) for good eye health is suggested by the fact that concentrations of this nutrient in the aqueous humor of the eyes is very high." He adds, "There is much evidence linking low intake of ascorbate to cataract formation...."

Research dating back to 1935 by Dr. Monjukowa found that patients with cataracts had a low level of vitamin C in their blood plasma. He concluded that deficiencies in vitamin C were not the result of the disease, but rather the cause of the cataract formation.

Treating The Cause, Not The Symptom!

Instead of treating the symptoms with eyedrops or the like, researchers are finally recognizing the benefit of correcting the problem; that is, giving your body the nutritional supplement it lacks.

In a study conducted by Dr. D.S. Devamanoharan of the Department of Ophthalmology at the University of Maryland, intake of vitamin C (ascorbate) has clearly proven effective in treating cataracts.

Dr. Passwater of the University of Western Ontario, found that daily supplements of 400 IU of vitamin E and 300 IU of vitamin C is a practical treatment against cataracts. The study concluded that a treatment combining both vitamin E and vitamin C supplements has an even greater effect on cataract prevention.

A report in the *American Journal of Clinical Nutrition* by Dr. S.B. Varma explained similar findings. Dr. Varma stated, "the cataractogenic effect...can be thwarted by nutritional and metabolic antioxidants such as ascorbate, vitamin E and pyruvate. These agents, therefore, may be useful for prophylaxis or therapy against cataracts."

Vitamin E (tocopherol) has also tested effective in preventing cataract formation according to a report in the *Journal of Nutrition* by Dr. G. Bunce. In a study of pregnant rats, Dr. Bunce found that a diet deficient in vitamin E resulted in cataracts in one-fifth of the newborns. Other scientific findings reported by Dr. W. Ross in the *Journal of Experimental Eye Research* indicates that vitamin E also delays or reduces the risk of cataracts.

50 To 70% Reduction In Cataract Risk!

The results of a serum analysis confirmed that a very high percentage of patients with cataracts had low levels of vitamin E and C. In a recent Canadian study, reported in the *American Journal of Nutrition*, Dr. J. Robertson concluded that "consumption of supplementary vitamins C and E may reduce the risk of senile cataracts by about 50 to 70 percent."

These findings have significant implications, considering there are more than one million cataract operations being performed annually in the United States. According to a recent report by the Associated Press, government guidelines are encouraging eye doctors to consider alternatives to surgery. The U.S. government spends $3.4 billion on cataract surgery for Medicare patients each year.

Vitamin A–Ground Breaking Studies!

"Have you ever seen a rabbit with glasses?" Believe it or not, the question has more scientific significance than you may have imagined. In a study of rabbits, scientists have uncovered a link between the nutrient beta-carotene (which is converted to vitamin A in the liver) and good eye sight. Dr. D.M. Geller, of the Department of Ophthalmology at Mount Sinai School of Medicine, found that carotene and vitamin E prevented cataracts in rabbits.

Clinical trials have also uncovered the value of vitamin A in the treatment of an assortment of other eye disorders. Harvard researchers have reported that vitamin A may be the first successful treatment of retinitis pigmentosa (RP). RP is an inherited disease characterized by degeneration of the retinal function. According to the results of a study by Dr. E.L. Berson of the Berman-Gund Laboratory for the Study of Retinal Degenerations at Harvard Medical School, vitamin A therapy will help alleviate the disorder and allow people with RP keep their vision longer.

While this is not a cure, it provides good news for the one-in-4,000 people who suffer from the disease. However, be advised that researchers warn against self-treatment without the supervision of an eye doctor.

According to the *Textbook of Anatomy and Physiology*, a deficiency in vitamin A is also linked to night blindness, softening of the cornea and conjunctivitis (pinkeye). Dr. G. Milkie reported at the annual meeting of the American Academy of Optometry that beta-carotene can help prevent blindness as well as corneal lesions. Milkie also commented that lack of zinc oxide deters the eyes ability to adjust in darkness. Dr. K. Seetharam Bhat, an Indian researcher, found that zinc and copper may be associated with the formation of cataracts.

Health Treatments From The Past

The latest findings about "new" treatments often come from remedies that have been used for centuries. Goldenseal root (*Hydrastis canadenis*), used by Native American Indians, can significantly reduce inflammation of the eye and treat eye infections. Dr. Gibbs and Dr. Nandkarni in separate studies confirmed that the herbs have potent antibiotic and antiseptic qualities.

An extract from the eyebright plant (*Euphrasia officinalis*), a European plant that grows wild, has been used for 2,000 years for treatment of eye infections. In the book, *The Scientific Validation of Herbal Medicine*, Dr. Mowrey states, "Most cases involve sore and/or inflamed eyes in which there is considerable stinging and irritation associated with watery-to-thick discharges, or conjunctivitis (pinkeye). The herb may help relieve other symptoms that often accompany inflamed eyes, such as a runny nose, earache and sneezing. Science has been remiss in not investigating this herb."

Researchers have now backed up the treatment with scientific evidence that eyebright alleviates sensitivity to the light and soothes acute and chronic inflammation of the eyes. Eyebright may be used as a topical eyewash or compress. For best results with topical applications, the whole herb should be dried before being used. For relief of conjunctivitis and blepharitis, it should be taken orally.

Sources Of Substances Mentioned
In This Chapter:

Billberry anthocyanosides, ascorbate (vitamin C), tocopherol (vitamin E), beta-carotene (vitamin A), goldenseal root and eyebright are available in many vitamin and health food stores.

Gero Vita Laboratories, a nutrition company, has developed *Ocu-Max*, an oral daily supplement, which contains many of the substances mentioned in this chapter in addition to other ingredients. The supplement contains tocopherol (vitamin E), carotene (vitamin A), ascorbate (vitamin C), zinc oxide, vanadium, cuberic oxide, selenium, molybenum, eyebright and bilberry extract. Gero Vita International, Dept. Z101, 2255-B Queen Street East #820, Toronto, Ontario M4E 1G3, Canada, or call (800) 825-8482.

BioEnergy Nutrients sells a product guaranteed to contain 25% anthocyanosides (bilberry extract). Write to them at 6395 Gunpark Drive, Ste. A, Boulder, CO 80301-3390. (800) 627-7775.

15

Preventing Heart Disease, High Cholesterol And High Blood Pressure

The facts are that heart disease is the cause for 1.25 million heart attacks each year in the United States, according to the U.S. Surgeon General's Report on Nutrition and Health. Two thirds of these attacks occur in men; annually 500,000 people die.

Why Do Heart Attacks Happen?

A heart attack occurs when the small blood vessels supplying the heart muscle are blocked. Blockage is a result of a chemical reaction very similar to the one that causes meat and butter to become rancid. It plays an important role in atherosclerosis–the development of artery-clogging plaque. Low-density lipoproteins (LDLs)–the so-called 'bad' lipoproteins –carry 60 to 80 percent of the cholesterol in the blood," according to the article "Hearty Vitamins" in *Science News*.

Studies over the past decade suggest that the adherence of fatty deposits to artery walls is the result of chemical modification of LDL through the process of oxidation (when LDLs join with oxygen).

This oxidation occurs when a cell called a macrophage consumes oxidized LDLs, creating "foam" cells. These foam cells adhere to arterial walls and collect atherosclerotic plaque. This plaque is what blocks the small blood vessels which supply the heart muscle.

Balanced Diets And Drug Therapy May Not Be Enough!

Dr. J. M. Ellis, in his book *Free of Pain*, states, "Most doctors and dieticians advise patients to eat a balanced diet to get all bodily nutrients needed." He wonders why then do most Americans end life with yellow and stiff blood vessels lined with hardened material.

Decreasing fat alone can be helpful because substances in fat can increase productivity of free radicals, causing atherosclerosis, resulting in critical nervous system, liver and kidney damage, as well.

When the processed-food industry and medical professionals urged Americans to stop eating butter and saturated fats and start eating margarine, they did not realize its danger to good health. According to Dr. A.I. Fleischman in "Titrating Dietary Linoleate To In Vivo Platelet Function In Man" from the *American Journal of Clinical Nutrition*, margarine actually increases the risk of a blood clot closing an artery (thrombosis).

In Heart Alert, Dr. A. Helgeland reported in "Treatment of Mild Hypertension: A Five-Year Controlled Drug Trial: The Oslo Study" in the *American Medical Journal*, that "diuretics (water pills) can cause all kinds of problems with heart patients."

Dr. S. A. Rogers, reports in his book, *Tired or Toxic?*, "In the Oslo Heart Trial, diuretics tripled mortality. Diuretics and some prescription antiarrhythmic drugs can actually cause arrhythmias" (irregular rhythm of heart's beating) "and heart attacks by washing magnesium, potassium and other nutrients needed for heart function out in the urine."

Nutritional Supplements May Prevent Heart Disease!

The research of Joseph G. Hattersley, as reported in an article in *Heart Alert,* states that heart attacks and strokes (caused by blockage of blood vessels supplying the brain) have declined since 1965. "Many doctors feel this is due to America's fad of taking vitamins."

Hattersley also discovered deaths resulting from coronary disease dropped by more than 42 percent (300,000 fewer deaths in 1986) than expected. While medical care (drug therapy and surgical intervention) and lifestyle changes (balanced diets, exercise and quitting smoking) have played a role, so has the use of nutritional supplements.

How Cayenne Pepper Capsules Can Help You Fight Heart Disease!

In Richard Quinn's book, *Left For Dead*, Quinn tells about his experience of having a heart attack, followed by bypass surgery which was supposed "to make me as good as new but didn't." He states his cardiologist said, "There is nothing more we can do."

Determined not to be counted as a death by heart attack statistic, he followed the advice of a friend and purchased cayenne pepper. He filled several capsules and swallowed them. He reported that the next morning he arose and shoveled four feet of wet snow off his 28-foot porch roof.

Thirteen years later, Quinn was still healthy. He studied the medicinal properties of other well-known herbs and began a company called Heart Foods. He started helping people with his inexpensive, safe cayenne capsules. However, the Federal Drug Administration (FDA) began harassing businesses that were selling his products.

How Cayenne Pepper
Prevents Heart Disease!

Cayenne capsules probably treat cardiovascular disease by acting as a general stimulant and reducing cholesterol buildup. Studies with albino rats show that capsaicin (which gives cayenne pepper its hotness) increases the change of cholesterol to bile acids. Cayenne lowers the blood cholesterol level by binding cholesterol and bile acids in the intestinal tract, which then is excreted.

Bile, which aids in digestion, is the bitter yellow, or greenish fluid secreted by the liver and found in the gall bladder.

Cayenne capsules can also aid in the cure of gastric ulcers, depression, chronic fatigue or prostration. The strength of the cayenne pepper is measured in heat units. Taken in gelatin form, cayenne does not burn the mouth. Cayenne based formulas are sold in health food and vitamin stores.

New Findings Question Aspirin
Therapy For Heart Disease!

"Taking an aspirin every day to help cut your risk of heart disease is no longer the way to go for many people," reports the American Heart Association (AHA). According to the AHA statement, aspirin therapy should only begin with a doctor's recommendation.

A special report issued by Dr. Valentin Fuster of Harvard Medical School and Dr. Charles Hennekens, lead investigator of the Physicians' Health Study (a study to test the effects of aspirin on heart disease), examined the benefits and dangers of using aspirin therapy. This report concludes that only a small segment of the population should be taking aspirin daily to prevent heart attacks."

How Aspirin Works!

Aspirin does not permit platelets in the blood to clump together to form blood clots that can block the vessels. Aspirin only helps in preventing blood clots which lodge in already narrowed arteries. According to the AHA, aspirin does not reverse the "hardening" caused by atherosclerosis.

Aspirin Has Negative Side Effects!

Dangerous side effects of using aspirin therapy affect patients with kidney disease, liver problems, peptic ulcers, gastrointestinal problems and bleeding disorders.

The AHA recommends prudent use of aspirin therapy in middle-aged or older men with obvious risk factors for heart attack. Other heart disease patients should seek their physician's advice regarding the use of aspirin therapy.

Natural Aspirin Substitute Works Like New Clot-Busting Drugs!

Clots formed in arteries are composed largely of protein. A protein mesh of fibrin encases each clot which includes fats and cholesterol. "Protease," or bromelain, is an enzyme extracted from the pineapple plant which breaks down those proteins.

The new clot-busting drugs Streptokinase (or Streptase) and urokinase dissolve 70 percent of the clots in heart patients by breaking down fibrin.

Bromelain, a non-prescription nutrient, also breaks down the fibrin mesh encasing clots of fats and cholesterol as reported in several medical journals, including the *Archaeological International Pharmacodyn*, the *Medical Hypothesis* and *the Journal of International Academy of Preventive Medicine.*

Bromelain may also "clean" plaque from arteries before a problem occurs. In a study of the aortas of rabbits, bromelain broke down the plaque present. It appears to keep clots from forming originally. This natural aspirin substitute prevents the production of prostaglandins. Some of these prostaglandins make cells sticky. Stickiness enhances clot formation.

L-Carnitine Strengthens Your Heart!

Studies have shown the importance of L-carnitine in strengthening the heart, relieving chest pain and lowering blood fat levels. This substance occurs naturally in many foods and also is available in health food and vitamin stores.

According to the *New England Journal of Medicine*, carnitine is essential for fatty acid oxidation and energy production. Severe and chronic L-carnitine deficiency may be associated with various cardiac problems: cardiomegaly, congestive heart failure and cardiac arrest. Ninety-five percent of the carnitine found in the body appears in cardiac and skeletal tissue.

How Carnitine Works!

According to *The Life Extension Update* newsletter, carnitine lowers triglyceride levels and elevates HDL cholesterol (the good cholesterol). Other benefits of using a carnitine supplement are that it reduces blood fat levels, "improves heart arrhythmias, increases stress resistance, lessens electrocardiogram abnormalities and improves exercise tolerance."

Heart attack victims benefit from intravenous administration of carnitine. This is because the coronary arteries dilate and a decrease damage to the heart muscle. The *Physician's Desk Reference*, states carnitine improves "tolerance of ischemic heart disease, myocardial insufficiencies and elevated blood fats."

Preventing Heart Attacks And Strokes With Fish Oil!

Reported studies have shown the American diet is considerably low in omega-3 oil. Fish oil containing omega-3 fatty acid has been found to actually reduce the LDL cholesterol and raise the good HDL cholesterol.

Abnormalities in heartbeat, kidney malfunction, fatty degeneration of the kidneys and liver, brain damage, elevated cholesterol, triglycerides and high blood pressure have all been shown to be caused by a deficiency in omega-3 oil.

One or two tablespoonfuls of an oil rich in omega-3 can be an important part of a healthy diet, especially if fish is not eaten regularly.

Results Of Taking Omega-3 Oil Show Success!

Dr. Dattilo advised people to eat fish which have omega-3 in his article in the *Journal of Cardiopulmonary Rehabilitation*. Eicosapentaenoic acid (EPA) is an excellent source of omega-3 oil. EPA comes from cold-water marine fish such as halibut, salmon, mackeral and albacore tuna.

EPA in the diet can result in a higher HDL to LDL ratio and much lower blood cholesterol and triglycerides. Fish oils may also keep blood cells from sticking together on the arterial wall, thereby reducing tryglycerides.

Coenzyme Q-10 Combats Heart Disease!

In a six-year study of patients with cardiomyopathy (a severe form of heart disease), a 75 percent survival rate was achieved when patients took coenzyme Q-10 (CoQ10). In comparison, patients receiving conventional therapy achieved only a 25 percent survival rate.

Heart disease patients often are deficient in CoQ10 and require more of it. CoQ10 may improve the strength of the heart muscle tissue, preventing congestive heart failure.

CoQ10 Deficiency Causes Heart Attacks!

In his article, "Coenzyme Q-10: The Nutrient of the 90's," Dr. R. A. Passwater explains CoQ10' s function in the production of energy in heart cells. He states that a number of heart attacks may result from a deficiency in CoQ10. According to Dr. Passwater, CoQ10 is present in most foods people eat, but it can't survive food processing and storage.

In 1957, CoQ10 was isolated by researchers who found it was a necessary nutrient for the body's cells. Since then the clinical value of CoQ10 has been demonstrated in the treatment of cardiovascular disease, angina, heart failure, hypertension and other serious disorders.

75% Of Heart Patients Can Benefit From CoQ10!

Dr. Karl Folkers, the discoverer of vitamin B6 and the father of CoQ research, believes CoQ deficiencies may be the major cause of heart disease.

Several heart patients at the Methodist Hospital of Indiana, who were given only days to live with traditional medications, had CoQ supplements added to their diets. Seventy percent survived for one year and 62 percent were alive after two years. Their cardiac functions improved, and they showed decreased difficulty in breathing and less fatigue. The symptoms of congestive heart failure present before using CoQ supplements disappeared after the CoQ treatment.

Other such studies have been conducted, with similar results, at the following institutions: Scott and White Clinic; Texas A & M; University at Temple, Texas; Kitasato University School of Medicine in Kanagawa, Japan; University of Bonn in West Germany; Municipal Hospital in Aarhus, Denmark; plus many other institutions around the world.

Dr. Folkers has studied patients with severe heart arrhythmias. He has shown these irregular heart beats were a direct result of a lack of CoQ. His research showed that the use of CoQ reduced or totally eliminated five of six patients' arrthythmias.

Millions Take CoQ10 As Nutritional Supplement!

According to Dr. Passwater, millions of people worldwide take CoQ10 supplements to counter heart disease, high blood pressure, aging and weakened immunity, as well as other conditions.

More than 12 million Japanese are taking daily doses of CoQ10, which was prescribed by their physicians to prevent and treat heart and circulatory diseases, reports Dr. G. L. Hunt in his article, "Coenzyme Q10: Miracle Nutrient?", printed in *Omni* magazine.

Heart attack victims in a Belgian study at the Free University of Brussels increased cardiac output and heart muscle strength after taking 100 mg daily for 12 weeks. Normally, heart muscle deterioration follows a heart attack. When CoQ was withdrawn, the previous benefits it produced, declined to the levels before CoQ treatment.

Vitamin B Lowers Dangerous Levels Of Homocysteine (HCY)!

HCY is a toxic amino acid derived from pasteurized cow's milk and red meat. It is a major cause of blood vessel disease (arterial lesions), according to Dr. K. S. McCully in his article, "Homocysteine Theory: Development and Current Status" from *Atherosclerosis Reviews*.

As reported in an article in a recent issue of *Heart Alert*, Dr. A.J. Olszewski stated that supplements of vitamin B6, choline and folate (all B vitamins) can lower HCY by 32% in three weeks.

Fluoridated Water Causes
Increase In HCY!

Dr. J. Yiamouiannis in his book, *Fluoride: The Aging Factor*, reports that fluoridated water lowers thyroid activity, which in turn increases HCY (confirmed by Dr. K. S. McCully in his article in *Atherosclerosis Reviews*).

Deficiency In Vitamin B6
Increases Heart Disease!

Scientists reported that when experimental animals on high cholesterol diets were given large doses of vitamin B6, they did not develop arterial plaque. Dr. Passwater in his book, *The New Supernutrition*, points to confirmation of this fact in other research. Some researchers concluded that higher levels of vitamin B6 may be required for heart disease prevention.

Importation Of Vitamin B6
Increased Substantially!

The U.S. Department of Commerce reported that the importation of vitamin B6 increased 5,400 percent from the mid-1960s to the mid-1980s. This suggests the use of vitamin B6 might, in part, be responsible for the declining death rate from heart disease.

Ideal Lifestyle And Diet May Not Be Enough
To Prevent Heart Disease!

In a study of a Pritiken group of heart patients who were semi-vegetarians, committed to exercise, not smoking and using physician prescribed medications, 60 to 65 percent as many suffered heart attacks "as would have been expected." Dr. R. J. Barnard reported these results in his article, "Effects of an Intensive Exercise and Nutrition Program on Patients with Coronary Artery Disease" in the 1993 *Journal of Cardiac Rehabilitation*.

The results of the Pritikin study suggest that an ideal diet and lifestyle adopted in midlife may be assisted by nutritional supplements in preventing heart attacks.

Taking Vitamin B Supplements Prevents Heart Disease!

Dr. J. M. Ellis in his book, *Free of Pain*, suggests individuals should take "around 5 mg per day of vitamin B_6 throughout life, along with vitamin B complex, vitamin C and other nutrients."

Dr. Ellis recommends B_6 combined with other nutrients processed from raw food source material. He recommends six to 15 tablets of Cardio-Plus daily. Synthetic time-released B_6 has been reported to cause liver problems.

Heart Patients Using Iodine-Rich Supplements Suffer Fewer Heart Attacks!

Dr. B. O. Barnes in his book, *Hypothyroidism: The Unsuspected Illness*, reported patients taking "iodine-rich supplements (like kelp) had few heart attacks. Those who quit taking supplements had more heart attacks." Dr. Barnes discovered and helped correct functional hypothyroid conditions in the general public. His work in identifying hypothyroidism and developing the proper treatments to correct it is a major accomplishment.

The research of Dr. K. S. McCully, presented in his article on homocysteine theory in the 1993 *Atherosclerosis Reviews*, confirms Dr. Barnes's conclusions.

Dr. McCully explained that a functional hypothyroid condition will lower a person's ability to store magnesium, and thereby raising the homocysteine in one's blood causing arterial lesions.

Taking Vitamin C Supplements Reduces Death By Heart Disease!

According to the National Health and Nutrition Examination Survey, men and women who took regular vitamin C supplements had 25 and 45 percent lower coronary mortality rates, respectively, than those with a lower intake of the vitamin.

Vitamin C promotes, good health in several ways. It controls the conversion of cholesterol to bile acids; it helps lower high cholesterol; and it prevents free radicals from oxidizing cholesterol in water soluble environment, such as the blood stream. Vitamin C also prevents free radicals from damaging lipids.

Vitamin C enhances the ability of the prostaglandin to keep blood cells from sticking together. This vitamin also helps arteries to dilate. A daily dose of two to three grams of vitamin C can reduce platelet stickiness, preventing plaque buildup.

Individuals with diseases such as diabetes mellitus and hypertension are at an increased risk of coronary artery disease because their levels of vitamin C are reduced. The elderly and male subjects, plus those who smoke, have reduced levels of vitamin C, increasing their risk of heart disease, according to *Clinical Pearls News*.

Magnesium And Tryptophan Deficiencies Cause Heart Attack Deaths!

Research has proven that some 20% of deaths from heart attacks are a result of coronary artery spasms triggered by deficiencies in magnesium and tryptophan. Tryptophan is obtained from protein rich foods.

Everyone Needs Cholesterol!

Cholesterol is a modified fat called a sterol, which is waxy, not oily or fatty. It doesn't dissolve easily in water or the blood stream. Cholesterol is made by the liver and smaller amounts are manufactured by the small intestine and individual cells throughout the body.

Cholesterol is important because it is used by every cell in the body to construct protective cell membranes. It acts as a barrier against substances trying to enter or leave the cell. It also supplies a protective barrier for the skin.

How Does Cholesterol Help Protect The Skin?

Cholesterol in the skin prevents certain liquids from penetrating the body and keeps water from leaving the body too quickly. The body loses only 10 to 14 ounces of water per day through evaporation, thanks to cholesterol.

Cholesterol helps provide the basis for steroid hormones produced by the adrenal glands, the ovaries and the testes. It also helps make vitamin D.

About 80 percent of cholesterol is used by the liver to help produce bile salts, which are stored in the gall bladder and used to aid in digestion and absorption of dietary fat.

How Much Cholesterol Does The Body Produce Daily?

Between 1,500 mg and 1,800 mg of cholesterol are produced by the body everyday. But only between 200 mg and 800 mg daily comes from the average American diet.

Blood Cholesterol Affected Little
By Dietary Intake Of Cholesterol!

In a *Federal Proceedings Abstract*, Dr. Slater reported that dietary cholesterol has only a slight effect on blood cholesterol levels in his article, "Effect of Dietary Cholesterol on Plasma Cholesterol, HDL Cholesterol and Triglycerides in Human Subjects."

This study was further confirmed in the famous Farmington study of 437 men and 475 women as reported by Dr. Gordon in "High Density Lipoprotein as a Protective Factor Against Coronary Heart Disease: The Farmington Study," published in an issue of the *American Journal of Medicine*. Dr. Gordon found no correlation between dietary intake of cholesterol and blood serum cholesterol.

How Does Cholesterol Work
In The Blood Stream?

UCLA and Harvard Medical School physicians and researchers offer this explanation. Low-density capsules of cholesterol are carried through the blood stream. These capsules are made up of apoproteins. Low-density lipoproteins (LDLs) move cholesterol from the liver to the heart and throughout the entire body. High LDL cholesterol levels mark a greater risk of heart attack.

High-density lipoproteins (HDLs) combine with cholesterol in the bloodstream and return it to the liver. In the liver, cholesterol is broken down. This is how HDLs can reduce the cholesterol buildup on an artery wall. Low levels of HDL have been associated with high risk of atherosclerosis.

In the July 1993 issue of *Science Journal*, medical geneticist Aldons Lusis, one of the five UCLA scientists who conducted research which was sponsored by the National Institutes of Health, explained the discovery of the apoprotein, apo A. Apo A II causes heart disease in mice. Mice given a low-fat diet had a "higher incidence of heart disease if that specific HDL protein was present." In other words, one of the proteins in the so-called good HDL cholesterol may not be so good. It is too early to determine "what foods promote high levels of good HDL cholesterol or lower levels of bad HDL cholesterol."

Many Factors Cause Atherosclerosis Resulting In 750,000 Deaths Annually!

No one single factor causes atherosclerosis. Cholesterol is just one of many factors affecting atherosclerosis. Other factors include: saturated animal fats, unsaturated fats, high blood pressure, age, heredity, smoking, insulin and hormones.

While cholesterol has been found in the plaque of clogged arteries, something must damage the arteries before the particles of cholesterol, calcium and blood fats can accumulate there.

Fats Affect Cholesterol!

Saturated animal fats raise blood cholesterol levels by oxidizing, and thereby creating free radicals, which inflame arterial walls. Saturated animal fats make blood cells stick together, causing reduced blood flow. This causes blood cells to clump and stick to artery walls. These clumps become receptacles for calcium and cholesterol deposits, thereby causing atherosclerosis.

Some vegetable and fish oils lower cholesterol levels and are antioxidizers neutralizing free radicals.

Blood Vessels And High Blood Pressure Affect Cholesterol Levels!

Blood vessels absorb nutrients and act as filters. Fat, carbohydrates and proteins are passed into the bloodstream and carried to different organs for storage or for immediate use. Some fat particles can't dissolve and may accumulate and form a plaque or blockage.

High blood pressure can trigger a rupture or hemorrhage in the tiny blood vessels that supply different layers in the artery walls. Fat circulating in the blood is released and accumulates in these areas.

Tiny arteries supplying the heart muscle are subjected to tremendous amounts of stress. Blocking these arteries leads to heart attacks.

Age, Heredity And Hormones Affect Cholesterol Levels!

Age affects the resiliency of arteries, resulting in the brittleness of arteries caused by calcium, cholesterol and other particles.

Heredity affects the incidence of atherosclerosis. and can affect mortality rates. Family histories should be examined so people can compensate for certain inherited weaknesses.

Also, hormones play a role. Estrogen protects women until menopause. This explains why atherosclerosis is so very common in men, who don't have the added hormonal protection.

Unique Case: Helen Boley Has Highest HDL Ever Recorded!

Scientists weekly draw a vial of the 61-year-old Mrs. Boley's blood, which is then rushed to the National Heart, Lung and Blood Institute in Bethesda, Maryland. Her blood is studied to learn how her body handles high- and low-fat diets, according to Dr. Kotulak in a 1991 report. Her HDL level is nearly five times higher than normal.

Her physician, Dr. William Harris, who heads the lipid laboratory at the University of Kansas Medical Center, says "She's preventing oxidation damage like crazy. Her arteries are probably squeaky clean."

Helen Boley is an example of genes or heredity affects body cholesterol levels. Researchers continue to learn how her HDL affects cholesterol levels.

Gene Therapy Helps Cholesterol Disorder!

According to an article, "Gene Therapy For Cholesterol Disorder," in *Science News*, success has been achieved in the first test of gene therapy to treat a rare, inherited form of high blood cholesterol.

The patient, a 29-year-old woman from Canada, has familial hypercholesterolemia. About 100 individuals in the United States have this ailment. It results in a genetic mutation which filters LDL cholesterol (so-called "bad" cholesterol) from the bloodstream.

James M. Wilson, of the University of Michigan Medical Center, announced the success of the treatment of an injection of genetically engineered liver cells, which lowered the LDL cholesterol in the patient from 500 milligrams per deciliter to 325 milligrams per deciliter. Even though the lowered level is still more than twice the healthy amount, the researchers believe further use of LDL cholesterol-lowering drugs will be beneficial, but some question their long-term use.

Study Proves Vitamin E Supplements Prevent Heart Disease!

As reported in *Science News*, a study of 24 men aged 25 to 70, some who were healthy, and others being treated for coronary artery disease, were split into two groups. One group took soybean-oil capsules for three months. The other group took similar capsules containing 800 international units (I.U.s) of vitamin E–80 to 100 times the recommended daily allowance of the body's premier antioxidant.

Researcher Dr. Ishwarlal Jialal, of the University of Texas Southwestern Medical Center, Dallas, and his co-worker, Scott Grundy, withdrew blood from each volunteer in the study preparing extracts of their LDLs. The LDLs have been subjected to conditions that foster oxidation.

At first, little difference was noted between the test groups. At 12 weeks, tocopherol (vitamin E) concentration was "4.4 times higher in the vitamin-supplemented group, according to a report in the *Journal of Lipid Research.*

The vitamin-supplemented test group had half the oxidative damage of LDLs. These men continued to be less susceptible to the oxidative process for the continuation of the study.

Taking Vitamin E Reduces Bad Cholesterol!

In *Science News,* Dr. Jialal said, "This is the first study to clearly show in a large number of patients that vitamin E has something to do with LDL oxidation."

Daniel Steinberg, of the University of California, San Diego, said, "The Dallas study clearly shows the protective effect (of antioxidant vitamins on LDLs). What we don't know is the degree of protection needed to have an impact on the atherogenic process."

Steinberg headed an antioxidant and atherosclerosis workshop at the National Heart, Lung and Blood Institute. Steinberg believes there is reasonably strong evidence that oxidation can aid atherosclerosis and antioxidants can slow plaque deposits in animals.

A Swedish study was discussed by Jan Regnstrom of the King Gustaf Vth Research Insitute in Stockholm and his colleagues in May 16, 1993 issue of the medical journal, *Lancet.*

Regnstrom concludes, "LDL susceptibility to oxidation would need to be taken into account as an important risk factor for coronary heart disease." Vitamin E is an antioxidant and improves the ability of oxygen to be absorbed into body tissue.

New Vitamin A, C And Beta-Carotene Trials To Start!

Several researchers, including Steinberg, plan to start trials to find evidence of boosting LDL oxidant defenses in people using combinations of vitamin E, vitamin C and beta carotene. Cigarette smokers will be included in the study because of the benefits they will receive.

Eat More Fiber To Lower Cholesterol Naturally!

According to an article in *Atherosclerosis*, Americans consume the least amount of fiber and have the highest heart disease rate in the world.

Fiber lowers cholesterol levels by increasing the amount of cholesterol excreted in daily bowel movements, as well as reducing the amount of cholesterol secreted by the liver. Fiber alters the type of bacteria in the colon.

Oats, Oat Bran, Metamucil And Guar Gum Are Worthwhile!

Oats and oat bran have been found by researchers at the University of Kentucky and the V.A. Medical Center to reduce LDL levels over 20% in 11 days, as reported in the *American Journal of Clinical Nutrition*.

Psyllium and Metamucil have shown that they can cause cholesterol to drop in two weeks. After eight weeks, total cholesterol was decreased by 25 percent, LDL cholesterol levels dropped 20 percent and the LDL/HDL ratio decreased from 3.2 to 2.6. The results of this study, as reported at an annual meeting of the Federation of American Societies for Experimental Biology, or psyllium indicated patients consumed one 3.4 gram packet of sugar-free Metamucil three times daily.

Guar gum (made from the guar plant of Texas, Mexico, Pakistan and India) can lower cholesterol levels as much as 25 percent. Guar gum products, such as Bio-Guar, a capsule, and Thera-Guar, a drink, are available in health food and vitamin stores.

Vitamin B3 (Niacin) Is A Cholesterol Reducer!

One of the least expensive natural alternatives to help lower cholesterol is niacin. According to a study published in the *Journal of Angiology*, only three grams of niacin a day reduced cholesterol levels 26% in just two weeks.

Taking the vitamin on a full stomach and in small doses can reduce possible flushing and itching side effects, reports an article in the *American Journal of Clinical Nutrition*. However, niacinamide, which works just as well, will not produce these side effects.

Vitamin C And Chromium Effectively Lowers Cholesterol!

Vitamin C, in doses as low as 500 mg to 1000 mg daily, was reported to significantly lower LDL cholesterol levels, according to the *American Journal of Clinical Nutrition* article.

Further evidence of vitamin C's cholesterol effect was mentioned in a 1984 issue of *Lancet* and the *Yearbook of Nutritional Medicine*.

Chromium, in the form of brewer's yeast (about 2 1/2 teaspoons daily), used by patients over an eight week period reduced serum cholester levels from over 240 mg to under 220 mg. HDL levels rose.

Under the direction of Dr. J.C. Elwood at the State University of New York, Upstate Medical Center at Syracuse, a study reported success using chromium. Subjects started with total cholesterol/HDL ratio averaging 5 and after the study, the ratio fell to 3.9. Anything above 4.5 is not acceptable for good cardiac health. The administration of one-half the previous dosages of the initial study resulted in a continued decline in almost 80 percent of the patients.

While brewer's yeast is the best source of chromium, someone, who has difficulty taking it, can take in its place 100 micrograms of chromium in tablet form to achieve similar results.

Chromium Picolinate Is The Best Choice!

One reason 90 percent of Americans take in less chromium than is needed for normal health is that food manufacuturers process their food too much, especially grains. More than 80 percent of natural chromium has been removed.

Another reason is that as individuals eat simple sugars, their bodies excrete large amounts of chromium.

One form of chromium, chromium picolinate, seems to be a much more effective dietary supplement than most other forms of chromium.

Dr. Jeffrey A. Fisher reported, "There have been several tests in which elevated cholesterol, elevated triglycerides, and reduced HDL or the so-called 'good' cholesterol in non-diabetics have improved following chromium supplementation. Subjects who had the highest insulin levels tended to improve the most. Dr. Evans and his colleagues tested the ability of chromium picolinate to lower cholesterol. His were the best and most consistent results obtained: a seven percent decrease in total cholesterol and an eleven percent reduction in LDL cholesterol after only six weeks on 200 micrograms per day of chromium."

"The form of chromium chosen for use is important," according to Dr. Fisher. He advises to avoid chromium with chromium chloride because it is poorly absorbed. He urges use of chromium picolinate.

Beta-sisterol Blocks
Accumulation Of Cholesterol!

Beta-sisterol, a phytosterol commonly found in vegetables, prevents cholesterol from accumulating in the arteries. The beta-sisterol supplement, for those who do not want to change their diets, is best taken immediately prior to eating. Dr. Matson reported that beta-sisterol lowered cholesterol in people whose diets otherwise remained the same.

Charcoal Absorbs Cholesterol!

Activated charcoal acts like a filter absorbing cholesterol. It also absorbs other potentially toxic chemicals, as well as nutrients.

In 1991 Dr. Passwater reported in a Finnish study that seven grams of activated charcoal taken daily for a month lowered LDL cholesterol by 41 percent.

Hawthorn Berries Improves
Heart Health!

In Europe, tinctures of hawthorn berries are used to lower cholesterol level and also as a heart tonic. Studies report that they strengthen and balance the heart rhythms. This naturally grown berry has prevented and reduced cardiac arrhythmias and protected the heart against oxygen deficiency. A study of 6,000 German patients using this medicinal herb discovered it improved heart health.

Individuals with heart disease are encouraged not to exclude more modern heart therapies. But, patients can safely use the properties of hawthorn berries in conjunction with modern medical heart therapy. Use 20 to 40 tincture drops twice a day. Hawthorne berry tea, made with a teaspoon of hawthorn berries, can be used often.

Complex CL-3 Used Successfully To Lower Cholesterol!

Those who are underweight or who've recently lost weight have high levels of HDL in their blood stream. Dr. Hans Kugler tested this assertion by formulating Complex CL-3. This nutritive improves the body's ratio of HDLs to LDLs.

Dr. Kugler discovered, in a controlled study using Complex CL-3, that individuals showed weight reduction even though they continued their normal dietary habits. An added benefit was a significantly reduced cholesterol level.

All Components Of Complex CL-3 Are Natural!

The components of complex CL-3 include *Allium sativum* (which lowers serum cholesterol), campesterol, stigmasterol and beta-sitosterol. These substances are derived from plants and called "sterols."

Scientists have shown that these substances inhibit cholesterol absorption into the blood. One study found that using these plant sterols to supplement a meal decreased cholesterol absorption by up to 64%.

Finally, the last component is oat bran, a source of fiber and vitamin B6, prevents extensive water retention and may act as a natural appetite control.

Vitamin A Therapy Reduces Cholesterol!

In the *Medical Journal of Australia*, a report of a study of a group of patients who were given vitamin A along with vitamin D for a 10 year period. The results were that those treated with vitamins A and D had one-third less cholesterol than untreated patients. Treated patients were given 25,000 I.U. of vitamin A and 400 I.U. of vitamin D.

Proanthocyanidine (PAC) May Block Accumulation of Cholesterol!

At an scientific symposium in France, Dr. David White of the University of Nottingham, England, reported PAC as "a powerful, non-toxic anti-oxidant that may block the accumulation of cholesterol." PAC acted to prevent the oxidation of LDL in test tube experiments.

Decreasing LDL oxidation is important because LDL causes the formation of plaque in the veins. Plaque blocks arteries which can lead to heart and circulatory diseases. Dr. White presented authoritative research that PAC reduces conditions that lead to cholesterol and foam cell formation.

Medicago Sativa Prevents Increase In Blood Cholesterol!

Medicago sativa contains many important substances including saponins, many sterols, flavonoids, coumarins, alkaloids, acids, sugars, proteins and trace elements.

Saponins have prevented increases in blood cholesterol levels by 25 percent when high cholesterol diets were fed to monkeys, rats and rabbits, according the Dr. M. R. Malinow in the *American Journal of Clinical Nutrition.*

Lecithin Is Helpful!

Lecithin is a phospholipid found in some vegetable foods, such as soybeans. It is also found in egg yolks, but is saturated and does not have the benefits of vegetable-derived lecithin.

Two to three tablespoons of lecithin per day has been reported to lower LDL cholesterol level. In a UCLA study, 48 grams of lecithin (1-1/2 ounces) taken daily lowered the cholesterol level 22% in a two-year period.

Allium Sativum!

Dr. A. Bordia, in *Lancet* (A British medical journal) reported that *Allium sativum* lowered blood serum cholesterol levels in animal and human research.

Dr. Kamanna later reported that *Allium sativum* "caused a marked reduction" in serum cholesterol levels in experimental animals.

High Blood Pressure Warning!

The *Surgeon General's Report on Nutrition and Health* stated that hypertension affects 20 to 30 percent of the adult population, or approximately 40 million Americans. High blood pressure causes heart failure and stroke. High blood pressure is related to coronary heart disease and atherosclerosis as well as other disorders.

According to the Surgeon General's report, close to 73 percent of all Americans have had their blood pressure checked during the last six months.

Blood pressure is read by expressing the systolic (measured when the heart is pumping the blood through a vein or artery at its greatest speed and volume) and diastolic (measured when the heart is resting and no blood is being pumped). Blood pressure is the ratio between these two readings.

Normal blood pressure readings range from 110 (systolic)/70 (diastolic) to 140/90. Readings of 140/90 to 160/95 indicate borderline hypertension. Any pressure reading over 180/115 is extremely dangerous.

Know The Symptoms and Precursors Of High Blood Pressure!

Advanced signs of hypertension include headache, sweating, rapid pulse, shortness of breath, dizziness and vision disturbances. Another common precursor of hypertension is atherosclerosis. Atherosclerosis involves the thickening, hardening and loss of elasticity in the walls of the arteries. The arteries become obstructed with cholesterol and mineral plaque, making circulation of blood through the vessels difficult.

Garlic Causes Reduction In Cholesterol Affects Blood Pressure!

Garlic taken as a dietary supplement can reduce serum cholesterol, serum triglycerides and blood fats. According to Dr. R. Bakhsh's article "Influence of Garlic on Serum Cholesterol, Serum Triglycerides, Serum Total Lipids and Serum Glucose in Human Subjects," subjects took dosages of 40 grams of garlic for a week while eating a fat-rich diet. The previous week they ate the same fat-rich diet without garlic.

When the blood serum cholesterol levels were tested in the subjects after using the garlic, the cholesterol levels had dropped, compared to the results of the cholesterol testing when the patients ate just a fat-free diet without garlic.

Dr. K. Gannon confirmed Dr. Bakhsh's findings in his article, "The Almighty Garlic: Can It Check Cholesterol Too?" in the journal *Drug Topics*. Dr. Gannon said, "Research has shown that consumption of garlic may lower cholesterol and blood pressure as well as help prevent some types of cancer."

Deodorized garlic can be purchased in health food stores under the name of SPG—odorless, tasteless, powdered garlic capsules. Recommended dosages are one capsule 6 times a day. As blood pressure stabilizes, the dosage can be reduced.

Potassium Reduces Blood Pressure!

Potassium is the opposite of sodium (salt) and aids in balancing the amount of salt in the body so that the heart and blood pressure remain normal. Conditions known to deplete potassium from the body include excessive salt, prolonged diarrhea or vomiting, use of diuretics, alcohol, coffee and sugar. Cortisone-like medications and patients with digestive tract diseases may also register low potassium levels.

A recent study showed that taking 9,000 mg of potassium chloride a day could drop blood pressure five to 20 points.

Calcium has been found to lower blood pressure by relaxing the small muscles surrounding blood vessels and helping to excrete extra salt from the body. A University of Oregon study showed that 1,000 mg of calcium daily for eight weeks dropped blood pressure 10 points in over 40 percent of the study participants.

Increased Dietary Fiber Helps!

Because high fiber diets (as opposed to high sugar diets) require less insulin to aid in digestion, blood pressure levels can be affected. Insulin makes the body retain salt, which can raise blood pressure.

Eating or supplementing one's diet with increased amounts of fiber can lower blood pressure levels as much as 10 to 15 points.

Coenzyme Q10 And Magnesium!

Studies at the University of Texas, and in Osaka, Japan, have shown that supplementing one's diet with 45 mg to 60 mg of CoQ10 could lower blood pressure levels as much as 12 to 25 points.

In a recent study of 61 older men, magnesium has been shown to result in lower blood pressure readings, according to an article in the *American Journal of Clinical Nutrition*.

Normally magnesium is lost through normal body functions by perspiring. It also is lost because of stress, use of alcohol, diuretics and sugar.

The natural dietary sources of magnesium include fresh green vegetables, raw wheat germ, soybeans, figs, corn, apples and nuts rich in oil.

Those whose diets are not rich in these natural foods may use magnesium supplements. Researchers recommend taking 500 mg daily.

Also, injections of magnesium sulfate lower blood pressure safely. In one study, the incidence of second heart attacks was cut by 87 percent.

Vitamin E And Iron Necessary!

Vitamin E helps the heart muscle use oxygen, while iron increases the oxygen-carrying ability of the blood. This vitamin and mineral can aid in lowering blood pressure.

Because initial high doses of vitamin E may temporarily raise blood pressure, authorities recommend the Dl-alpha tocopherol acetate form of vitamin E. Doses of 200 I.U. to 1600 I.U. daily are recommended either during or right after a meal.

People with heart or circulation problems may take vitamin E in smaller doses. People with these conditions should start with 50 I.U. to 100 I. U. daily and gradually increase dosages. Dr. William Shute's book, *Vitamin E for Ailing and Healthy Hearts,* provides more information on this subject.

Taking Procyanidin (Pycnogenol) Decreases Blood Pressure!

According to the research of Dr. David White, University of the Nottingham, England, pycnogenol reduces cholesterol and foam cell formation.

Dr. G. Blazso, in his article "Oedema-Inhibiting Effect of Procyanidin" in the *Journal Acta Physiologica Academiae Scientiarum Hungaricae,* has also shown the effectiveness of procyanidin.

Dr. Blazso found in experiments with animals that "when administered intravenously, a dose of 35 mg/kg led to a slight decrease in blood pressure while doses of 50 to 100 mg/kg gave rise to a long-lasting reduction in blood pressure."

A single 100 mg supplement of pycnogenol may increase the health of the capillary wall membranes allowing them to absorb vitamin C and increase their resilliency. A single supplement of 20 mg of pycnogenol was shown to improve vascular sensitivity by 82%.

Alfalfa Cleans The Blood!

Besides having almost every vitamin and mineral known to man, alfalfa is also a valuable resource of "phytosterols." As previously mentioned, phytosterols have been shown to neutralize harmful cholesterols. According to a study by Dr. Genazanni, it also affects high blood pressure.

Based upon the scientific research outlined in this chapter, the following supplements may prevent or alleviate heart problems:

- Cayenne pepper
- Bromelain
- L-carnitine
- Omega 3 (fish oil)
- Coenzyme Q10
- Vitamin B$_6$
- Vitamin B$_3$
- Vitamin C
- Vitamin B
- *Medicago sativa*
- Lecithin
- Allium sativa
- Kelp
  (iron supplement)
- Magnesium
- Tryptophan
- Vitamin E
- Vitamin A
- Beta-carotene
- Metamucil
- Guar gum
- Garlic
- Potassium
- Calcium
- Brewer's yeast
  (chromium)
- Chromium picolinate
- Beta-sisterol
- Charcoal
- Hawthorn berries
- Complex CL-3
- Oat bran
- Vitamin D
- Procyanidin
- Alfalfa

Sources Of Substances Mentioned In This Chapter:

Most of the substances mentioned in this chapter are available from local health food and vitamin stores. The following are mailorder sources:

L-carnitine	Life-Extension International 1142 West Indian School Road Phoenix, Arizona 85013-9985
Bromelain	Vitamin Research Products 1044 Old Middlefield Way Mountain View, California 94043 1-800-877-2447

Cayenne capsules

Heart Foods
1-800-CAYENNE
1-612-724-5226

PEPTI-GARD, available from
Gero Vita, Dept. Z101
1-800-825-8482

Complex CL-3

Gero Vita International,
Dept. Z101,
2255-B Queen Street East #820,
Toronto, Ontario M4E 1G3, Canada,
(800) 825-8482.

Proanthocyanidin
(procyanidin)

Natural Vitamins
P.O. Box 1117
St. Augustine, Florida 28085

Pycnogenol
Alfalfa

Alfa Flour
P.O. Box 332
Wray, Colorado 30766
1-303-332-3124

16

A Strong Immune System Means Less Sickness, Less Doctors And Less Drugs!

The body's first line of defense in maintaining health, preventing illness and lessening and healing its effects is the immune system. Researchers, health-care professionals and the public are asking the same questions: Why are some people more able to resist illness than others? How do age, lifestyle and the environment affect us? What can we do to strengthen our immune systems BEFORE we become ill?

The immune system recognizes, reacts to and removes foreign substances from the body, both chemical (as in infections) or cellular (as in tumor growth). Strong immune function requires adequate production of certain cells manufactured throughout the body, especially in the thymus and bone marrow.

The lymphatic system also plays an important role in immunity from illness. Waste matter is drained from the tissues by the lymphatic vessels. Lymph fluid is then "treated" by the lymph nodes, destroying bacteria and other toxins. The lymph nodes also manufacture lymphocytes, which begin antibody production. The largest body of lymphatic tissue is the spleen.

When The System Fails!

When the protective capabilities of the immune system goes awry, the result can be an allergic reaction to substances. If the system fails, resistance may weaken and allow an immune deficiency disorders such as AIDS or cancer.

A gradual weakening of the immune system is believed to be part of the aging process. However, research has shown that supplementing the immune system in various ways can help us to resist some age-related illnesses. For example, Dr. J.S. Thompson wrote in the journal, *Clinical Geriatric Medicine* that the aging process includes T-cell defects as well as zinc and protein deficiencies.

Reduce Your Vulnerability To Illness!

Certainly, a healthy lifestyle and avoiding toxins in the environment as much as possible are valuable steps in keeping immune function at its peak. In addition, according to the U.S. Department of Agriculture Human Nutrition Research Center on Aging at Tufts University in Boston, "dietary manipulation of the immune system has been proposed as a practical approach to intervening in its age-related functional decline." Fortunately, there are some natural substances which have shown promising results in this area, both in the laboratory and in actual treatment.

Beta-Carotene Boosts Immunity!

Beta-carotene is processed by the body into vitamin A. Increased beta-carotene intake has been recommended to help prevent certain cancers. In the *American Journal of Clinical Nutrition*, Dr. R.R. Watson reported a study which demonstrated increased T cell production in a group of ten men and ten women given 30 mg or more of beta carotene per day for two months. Useful as an anti-oxidant, beta-carotene may possibly kill viruses, and has been shown to boost CD4 cell production. Vitamin A deficiencies are thought to result in increased vulnerability to infection.

Vitamin E Is Valuable For The Elderly!

A recent study by Dr. S.N. Meydani in the *American Journal of Clinical Nutrition* found that a group of people over age 60 showed increased immune system function when given 800 IU of vitamin E every day for thirty days. In this study, the subjects were also found to have increased production of Interleukin-II, which stimulates T-cell production and is under investigation for AIDS treatment.

At the U.S. Department of Agriculture's Human Nutrition Research Center on Aging at Tufts University, studies proved that supplementing the diets of elderly people with vitamin E for one month strengthened their immune systems.

Amino Acids Stimulate The Youth Gland–The Thymus!

Arginine is an amino acid, which has been shown to increase the production of human growth hormone in the pituitary gland. Human growth hormone stimulates the thymus gland, which manufactures the T cells so vital to immune function. Levels of this hormone decline in the normal course of aging, and decreased amounts have been linked to the development of cancer, stroke and heart disease. When combined with another amino acid, lysine, researchers at the Italian National Research Centers on Aging in Acona, Italy, observed enhanced thymus functioning, and noted that thymus function can be stimulated to a "younger" level.

Natural killer cell development was observed in a group of young men, ages 21 to 34 who took 30 mg of arginine per day, according to a study published in the British medical journal *Lancet*. Natural killer cells are not manufactured in either the bone marrow or the thymus, and can destroy tumor and viral cells. This finding is significant in AIDS and cancer treatment, since T cells increased as well. Another study in the

Canadian Medical Association Journal noted that patients given arginine in conjunction with omega-3 fatty acid and RNA supplements had less postsurgical infection and shorter hospital stays.

In an effort to combat age-related immune system decline, researchers studied the effects of another amino acid, dimethylglycine (DMG). Reporting in *The Journal of Infectious Diseases*, Dr. C.D. Graber noted that DMG improved human immune response by enabling various substances to be circulated through the bloodstream more quickly. An additional study by Dr. E.A. Reap in the *Journal of Laboratory and Clinical Medicine* documented that "immunologic aberrations are well-known consequences of aging," and that "immune function in these various states might profit by treatment with a non-toxic immunomodulator, such as DMG."

New Benefits From Minerals!

Selenium was found to increase lymphocyte production in a study of elderly nursing home residents by Dr. A.M Peretz of the Department of Rheumatology and Physical Medicine at St. Pierre Hospital, Brussels, Belgium, in 1990.

Zinc encourages wound healing, aids thymus function and hormone activity. Dr. Castillo-Duran reported in the *American Journal of Clinical Nutrition* that giving zinc supplements to infants benefitted their immune defense ability.

Adequate iron is needed for red blood cell production. Copper is required to manufacture blood cells in the bone marrow. All of these functions are vital in resisting disease processes. In addition, iron, copper and zinc deficiencies can weaken immune system function. Dr. R.K. Chandra wrote in the *Journal of Dentistry for Children* that a lack of any of these minerals limits immunity.

Alkylglycerols May Prevent Tumors!

First discovered in 1922 in Japan, alkylglycerols are three natural substances produced in the liver. They also occur in breast milk, thus providing protection to newborns until their own immune systems develop.

In 1952 a Swedish physician, Astrid Brohult, M.D., discovered that children with leukemia increased their white cell counts when given bone marrow from newly slaughtered calves. Apparently, the marrow contained alkylglycerols. Later, Dr. Brohult found that patients with uterine or cervical cancer survived longer when given alkylglycerols.

Another potent and better-known source of alkylglycerols is shark liver oil, which has been used in Chinese medicine for over two thousand years to treat a variety of illnesses. Liver oil from certain species of sharks can contain up to a 90% concentration of alklyglycerols.

Alkylglycerols increase white blood cell (leukocyte) production. These cells contain antibodies, which are vital in warding off illness. Alkylglycerols have also been shown to slow white blood cell reduction during chemotherapy, to stimulate the immune system in viral infections and inhibit tumor growth in laboratory studies.

Phycotene And Echinacea!

Extracted from a combination of spirulina and dunaliella algae, phycotene contains numerous beta carotenes and vitamin E. In research studies at Harvard University, oral cancers in laboratory hamsters showed total remission in thirty percent of the animals tested, and partial remission in the remaining seventy percent. Joel Schwartz, M.D. of Harvard observed that phycocyanin-C (a component of phycotene) slowed tumor growth by creating a hostile environment around the tumor. In addition, phycotene increases TNF (a substance which destroys tumor cells) production which, when combined with interferon (another natural substance in the body which combats viral infections), tremendously increases immune function.

In use since the 1800s, echinacea has an antibiotic effect and increases the white blood cell count, thus strengthening the immune system. As D. Marley noted in *The Scientific Validation of Herbal Medicine*, "The herb acts effectively to close down one of the major routes of bug-invasion" by working with the hyaluronic acid found in human tissue to enable it to "stick together" and resist infection.

Co-Enzyme Q (CoQ)!

A naturally-occurring substance, CoQ has been shown to improve the immune function of existing cells. Unlike many drugs used today to fight immune system disorders, CoQ is relatively free of side effects and has been used along with conventional cancer chemotherapy. Long-term testing in the United States, Japan and West Germany has noted that the only side effect in varying doses is mild nausea, and that this rarely occurred.

Treatment with CoQ requires doses ranging from 30-100 mg per day. After ingesting CoQ, it is processed in the liver from CoQ 1-9 into CoQ 10. It is thought that this function of the liver retards aging and protects against disease.

CoQ has also demonstrated its value as an effective anti-oxidant/free radical scavenger. Oxidants, also known as free radicals, are substances produced in response to pollution, X rays, cigarette smoke and other toxins which are thought to damage healthy cells. CoQ's function would be to prevent these free radicals from affecting healthy cells, as well as to boost the immune system. CoQ is considered a vitamin, and correcting its deficiency could be helpful in curing illness.

All of the items discussed in this chapter are available at health food and vitamin stores. A good mail-order source is:

Bio-Energy Nutrients, Incorporated
6395 Gunpark Drive, Suite A, Boulder, Colorado 80301-3390.
Telephone (800) 553-0227.

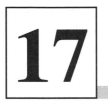

Cancer Prevention!

Cancer is a group of diseases having a common characteristic: uncontrolled multiplication of cells that crowd out healthy tissue, eventually shutting down vital body organs.

Since there are so many cancers which grow and travel at different rates of speed and attack different parts of the body, it is no wonder that no simple cause or cure can be identified. It is equally unsurprising that the cancers are not fully understood, although research is going on all over the world to identify causes, possible preventives and cures.

We know from ancient burial excavations and history that cancer has always been with us, the incidence of cancer has been increasing with the industrial era, coinciding with increasing longevity and an increasingly toxic environment. Cancer is right behind heart and circulatory failures as a leading cause of death.

How We Fight Cancer!

Of course, new technology has provided some of the means to identify and combat the effects of cancer by means of radiation, surgery and chemotherapy. None of these are without risk or harm to healthy tissue.

However, the advancement of chemical and physical analyses, together with formalized clinical trial techniques, have enabled researchers to take a look at alternative systems of medicine, as well as at our bodies' systems for fighting invaders such as cancer.

Researchers are asking what natural substances have benefits? How and why do they work? Can rare substances be synthesized? Can our own immune system be reinforced against cancers, as it has been against other dreaded diseases such as smallpox and polio?

Cancer Fighters Exist In Nature!

Cancer treatment is changing very quickly, and you are likely to find that some of the substances we mention in these pages that have not been included as part of conventional medical practice, are being explored by established medical scientists. An example: Taxol, of which two or three doses are produced from one western yew tree, is being tested in clinical trials because of its potential importance against breast and ovarian cancers.

Obviously there aren't enough western yews if Taxol proves to be effective and safe. Therefore synthetics are in development stage at Bristol Myers Sqibb Company and at Rhone-Poulenc Rorer Inc. in France. The National Cancer Institute is sponsoring clinical trials of Taxol, as well as evaluations of other substances.

Different Countries, Different Cancers!

The sciences of communication, statistics and epidemiology have taught us that there are vast differences in the incidence and types of cancers that strike the populations of various countries and continents. Obviously, the differences in environment and diet offer different dangers as well as protections. Some factors are well enough established (such as air pollution and DDT) to be the subject of protective legislation. Many others are in various stages of research.

As mentioned earlier, there is uncertain profit in establishing the curative powers of a natural substance; therefore, much of the research has been with small samples, or laboratory animals, or inferred from observation of available human subjects. An example of the latter is that Japanese women living in Japan have a fraction of the rate of breast cancer that prevails in the United States. When they come here to live, their rate of breast cancer approaches ours.

It is likely that promising research projects will benefit from support by non-profit enterprises such as the National Cancer Institute. And it can also be expected that to the extent natural substances can be synthesized, they will be patented and made available.

Sharks Are Immune To Cancer!

Another rare feature of sharks is that their skeletons are made of Cartilage. Cartilage has no blood vessels. In fact, it contains a protein that inhibits the development of blood vessels.

The rapid growth of cancerous masses requires that they have a matching growth in blood supply. A research team at Children's Hospital in Boston headed by Dr. Judah Folkman, working with various inhibitors, tried shark cartilage. They discovered that a tumor will stop growing at one to two millimeters if it doesn't have a blood supply.

The effectiveness of shark cartilage has been confirmed on laboratory animals at Massachusetts Institute of Technology (MIT), reported by Dr. Robert Langner in the *Journal of Biological Response Modifiers*. Dr. G. Atassi of the Institute Jules Bordet in Belgium, had the same results. The application of shark cartilage was by oral administration of dried cartilage.

Terminal cancer patients at the Centro Medico del Mar in Tijuana, Mexico. showed great improvement–40% to 100% reduction in tumor size–within the first 60 days of the study. At this site, the shark cartilage extract was administered in solutions, rectally and vaginally.

Shark cartilage has been standardized for research and therapy by Dr. William Lane. The cartilage is a by-product of sharks harvested for food in Costa Rica, where the product Cartilade is manufactured.

Although shark cartilage is not toxic and can be taken at the same time as any other cancer treatment, there are conditions under which it shouldn't be administered because new blood vessel growth is wanted: after a heart attack or stroke, during pregnancy, or in cases of lesions that won't heal.

Ginseng And Melatonin!

There are several kinds of ginseng, which have been used in numerous human and animal studies. In test tube studies in Japan, ginseng is said to have caused liver cancer cells to revert to normal form.

Melatonin, an inexpensive, non-toxic and non-prescription drug, has had a favorable effect on the immune system of laboratory animals. It appears to halt the progress of breast cancer, and even to cause tumors to regress. It is the subject of several current studies. Researchers are aware of its potential.

Colon Cancer: Eating To Prevent It!

There is general agreement, based on observation, that a diet rich in fruits, leafy vegetables and fiber protects against colorectal disease. To further refine this information, a group of researchers at Harvard Medical School, directed by Dr. Edward Giovannucci, found that folate (a B vitamin in leafy vegetables,) and methionine an amino acid found in high protein foods like fish and chicken protecti against colon polyps. Folate supplements give even greater protection, according to the *Journal of the National Cancer Institute.*

Consensus On Dietary Supplements!

Both traditional and alternative approaches to cancer prevention or therapy appear to accept the theory that cancer implies a breakdown or overload of the immune system. Many of the substances recommended to repair or stimulate the immune defenses are aimed at helping rid our bodies of the toxins we take in from the environment or from foods.

The Harvard group mentioned above examined the cancer statuses and diets of thousands of subjects in a long-term health study of nurses and physicians who volunteered to be followed over decades. Many studies confirm that superior health status, including lower occurrence of cancers, are associated with a healthy diet plus multi-vitamin and mineral supplements.

The head of the Cancer Research Institute at the University of Vienna, Dr. Heinrich Wrbe, has concluded that "dietary supplements can cut your risk of cancer by 50%." The exceptional health benefits of vitamin and mineral supplements have also been put forward in *Lancet*, the prestigious British medical journal.

Breast Cancer: How Is It Linked To Diet?

The Harvard Medical School study, previously mentioned, queried 1,439 female nurses who developed breast cancer, and found no link to dietary intake of fat, according to the *Journal of the American Medical Association*.

However, it is established that carcinogenic poisons such as DDT are stored in body fat for decades.

The extensive comparison of Japanese and American women points to a vast difference in fat intake. Body fat increases the level of estrogen, and high levels of estrogen are associated with breast cancer.

Breast Cancer Inhibitors
In The Japanese Diet!

The Japanese diet, unlike ours, is rich in fish, fiber, soy products and various seaweeds. The following substances, prominent in the Japanese diet, have been found in laboratory tests with animals to inhibit the growth of tumors.

Seaweed, especially Laminaria, was explored by Dr. Ichiro Yamamoto, because it is an ancient Chinese remedy. Extract of Laminaria appeared to cause regression of tumors in mice. The active ingredient is a polysaccharide that helps the body dissolve certain fatty substances, according to the *Japanese Journal of Experimental Medicine*.

Soybeans inhibit a protein digesting enzyme (protease) that is more abundant when there is a breast malignancy. Laboratory experiments showed that animals exposed to carcinogens developed tumors at nearly half the rate of the control group when they were fed soybean products.

The Japanese diet abounds in soybean dishes, such as miso soup and tofu. Selenium, an essential mineral, is four times more abundant in the Japanese diet than in ours, and it is believed to be effective in preventing and reducing breast tumors. Japanese studies have demonstrated that selenium, with other minerals and vitamins such as magnesium and ascorbic acid (vitamin C) inhibit the growth of breast cancer in laboratory rats. These studies were reported by Dr. A. Remesha in the *Japanese Journal of Cancer Research*.

War Against Cancer
Is Waged On Many Fronts!

With the incidence of the most prevalent cancers increasing, there is a great deal of investigative activity, with many conditions and substances being explored simultaneously. It is generally accepted theory that more than half of human cancers have environmental causes, such as smoke, ionizing radiation and toxic industrial chemicals, with most other carcinogens being ingested via food, water and air. It's even thought that some factors act only in combination to promote tumors. Dr. William Marcus of the Environmental Protection Agency points out that chlorinated tap water is associated with high rates of breast cancer. Is this a coincidence or another cause?

The National Cancer Institute is evaluating numerous studies that are exploring the effect of various substances and food supplements, such as those mentioned before and after this paragraph. Before continuing, we think it preferable to try to explain, at least superficially, the action of anti-oxidants in the cause of cancer.

Free Radical Oxidants And Anti-Oxidants!

You can see free radicals in action when oxygen in the air to combines with iron, which it "oxidizes" to form rust. Oxidation is going on in our bodies all the time, converting digested food to energy and new cells as we need them. Free radicals seek to combine, and will destroy any cell that they hit! Occasionally they alter the DNA structure somewhere in our bodies, so as to give a cell changing the instructions for reproduction. Such a cell may mutate (permanently change) via its offspring, and may not only deform, as in aging, but begin abnormally rapid reproduction.

It is the function of your immune system to send "killer" white blood cells and super oxide dimutase (SOD) to remove dangerous invaders. The task of your liver to remove harmful toxins and excrete them through the kidneys and intestines.

Many foods and supplements contain anti-oxidants that reinforce the cleansing functions of the immune system and the liver. This finding is reported in many publications, including for example, *Hematology/Oncology Journal* and in *The New Supernutrition* by Dr. Richard Passwater.

Synergy!

Certain anti-oxidants, when combined, enhance each other's potency, in an effect called "synergy"–working together for a result that each alone could not achieve.

For example, vitamins B_{12} and C together entirely prevented the growth of transplanted mouse tumors, reported in *Experimental Cell Biology* by Dr. Poydock.

The National Cancer Institute is funding dozens of studies exploring the efficacy of nutrients in cancer prevention. Among the anti-oxidants now recommended are beta-carotene plus vitamins C and E.

Although all the studies of anti-oxidants may not be completed, it seems like a good idea to adopt a protective diet that appears to work. Note that high levels of selenium are present in the diet of Asian peoples with low incidence of breast cancer. Dr. Passwater found that selenium works in synergy with vitamin E to prevent and reduce cancers.

Beta-carotene is thought to be especially protective against lung cancer, according to Dr. Passwater.

Vitamin C has long been promoted by Nobel laureate Dr. Linus Pauling, as protective against viruses and toxic chemicals, including those in food preservatives.

What is the anti-toxic effect? "Cured" foods such as ham and bacon and many others contain nitrates and nitrites for preservation. These combine, in the process of digestion, with amino acids to form nitrosamines, which are carcinogens. Vitamin C neutralizes the nitrates and nitrites. You can ingest vitamin C in fresh fruits and vegetables, and as supplement to your diet.

Vitamin E has a similar effect and is thought to reduce the level of substances that cause mutation of cells. Two separate studies of human subjects showed that in breast cancer patients and lung cancer patients, lower levels of vitamin E were present than in matched control subjects. These studies were reported in the *British Journal of Cancer* and in the *New England Journal of Medicine*.

Observed But Not Yet Understood!

Many elements that occur naturally in food are being studied because they have an observable connection with lowering cancer risk or growth, though their processes may not be fully understood. Some examples are:

Folic acid, a B vitamin, was observed to reduce lung injury from smoking by Dr. Douglas Hamburger of the University of Alabama.

Glutathione appears to bind with cancer causing toxins. In one study, this substance reversed liver cancer in rats which was reported in *Science Magazine*.

Cysteine neutralizes the chemicals that are the product of smoking and damage the immune system, according to Dr. Passwater.

Fish oil appears to prevent or stop the growth of some of the most common cancers: breast, pancreatic, and prostate.

Quercetin (found in broccoli, onion, squash and supplements) appears to be protect against colon cancer and enhances the strength of cell walls.

Magnesium has been reported to prevent cancer and enhances the strength of cell walls.

Some elements in food were found to be abnormally low in cancer patients. Are they ingested less or used up faster? Typical of these are zinc and stearic acid.

Lactobacillus acidophilus, found in acidophilus milk and yogurt, inhibits the formation of carcinogenic substances in the colon. This was reported was by Dr. B.R. Goldin in *Clinical Nutrition*.

Epigallocatechin gallate (EGCG), abundant in Asian diets, especially green tea, seems to be a factor in combating several specific types of cancer: colon, skin and lung. As reported during the proceedings of the American Chemical Society in 1991, EGCG reduces the rate of lung cancer in smokers.

DHEA–Low Levels In Cancer Patients!

Dehydroepiandrosterone (DHEA) is a hormone secreted by our adrenal glands. We secrete less as we grow older. Men with high levels of DHEA are half as likely to die of heart disease as men with low levels, according to Dr. Elizabeth B. Connor of the University of California at San Diego.

This same condition has been observed with cancer in other studies, and this substance is under such intense study that more health effects are emerging all the time. DHEA seems to have a stabilizing effect on all human body systems. It can help overweight people to lose, and underweight people to gain weight. As we have learned, body fat enhances the production of estrogen, which in turn can promote cancer growth.

DHEA Has Multiple Effects!

One of the principal investigators of DHEA, Dr. Arthur Schwartz of the Fels Research Institute of Temple University, has been working with mice. He found that DHEA helps burn off body fat and inhibit the growth of cancer cells. Other researchers have examined the effects of DHEA. Dr. Roger Loria of the Medical College of Richmond, Virginia, has demonstrated that it increases immune functions and helps fight viral infections.

There are many theories about how DHEA works to inhibit cancer growth. It appears to block growth of carcinogens. It may slow the productions of free radicals that are involved in the aging process and formation of abnormal cells. Another theory is that DHEA works like diet restriction, by inhibiting utilization of glucose, which is know to prolong life of laboratory animals.

A possible explanation is that by lowering body temperature (not burning glucose) the repair of DNA is enhanced, thus reducing the reproduction of mutated cells.

Many studies of DHEA are in process or in planning. It appears thus far that its effect varies with the cancer type, which can vary with age (hormonal status) even at a single site.

It has been observed that DHEA levels fall during serious illness and rise during exercise, which tends to confirm its association with well-being. Among those making this observation are Dr. E.D. Lephart, in the *Journal of Clinical Endocrinology Metabolism* and Dr. P.Diamond, reporting in the *European Journal of Applied Physiology*, among others.

Sources Of Substances Mentioned In This Chapter:

DHEA or its synthetic form is marketed for many diagnoses beside cancer: gout, cirrhosis, psoriasis and post-menopausal depression. It is sold in Europe as PROSTERONE or ASTENILE.

None of the numerous studies involving DHEA has indicated that it does harm. It is not widely available, possibly because no one has a stake in its distribution. Your pharmacist may be able to supply it. We know that it has been available by mail recently from:

Belmar Pharmacy
8015 West Alameda Ave. Suite 100
Lakewood, CO 80226
Phone 800-525-9473

College Pharmacy
833 North Tejon Street
Colorado Springs, CO 80903
Phone 800-749-2263

Other substances mentioned in this chapter:

Melatonin:
Life Extension Foundation
1-800-841-5433

Cartilade (Shark Cartilage):
Cartilage Technologies Inc.
222 Grace Church Street
Port Chester, N.Y. 10573

The following are usually available from vitamin and health food stores:

Alkyloglycerol
Ginseng
Folate supplements (folic acid)
Beta-carotene
Seaweed (Laminaria)
Soybean products, including miso and tofu
Fish oil
Glutathione
Cysteine
Quercetin

Epigallocatechin gallate (ECGC) is for professional experimental use only at this time, but it may be obtained by drinking Oriental green teas which are available in some health food stores and in Japanese or Chinese neighborhoods.

18

Answers To Ulcers, Digestion And Colon Problems!

If you were asked to name the group of related diseases for which the largest number of Americans are hospitalized each year, what would your answer be? Surely, most people are admitted into the hospital due to heart and lung ailments, you might answer. Or perhaps, you are certain that diseases related to the body's immune system are the cause for most Americans being hospitalized each year.

Surprisingly, according to *Bio/Tech News*, diseases of the digestive tract head the list of ailments that put Americans in the hospital. The statistics are particularly staggering. Nearly 100 million of us experience some form of reoccurring digestive disease, with 200,000 of us missing work per day.

All of these huge numbers point to an obvious problem. We are a nation ruled by its stomach (and other digestive organs), and apparently that battle is being won by the other side. A good strategist would tell you that the enemy must be studied to learn its strengths and weaknesses. After long years of study, scientists and doctors have found that the war we've been waging with prescription drugs may well be better won with more natural means.

Diseases Of The Digestive System Were Virtually Unknown Until This Century!

Two of the largest and most menacing of the players in the war are cancer and various ailments of the colon, rectum and digestive system which include constipation, appendicitis, diverticular disease, hemorrhoids, irritable bowel disease, ulcerative colitis, Crohn's disease, benign tumors and stomach ulcers. Evidence of these diseases hardly existed in the Western world a 100 years ago. This becomes even more telling when we look at certain non-Westernized cultures, like pre-World War II Japan and some parts of modern day Africa. These cultures show almost no evidence of the digestive diseases mentioned. The culprits do show up as soon as these societies become "Westernized"; that is, take on our diets.

Studies Began Early!

A handful of doctors in the United States, Great Britain, and working in Third World nations began to make the connection between a low fiber diet and the upsurge of digestive diseases as early as the 1920's. British physicians Dr. Arthur Rendle-Short, Dr. Robert McCarrison, and Dr. Arbuthnot Lane all drew attention to the need for a high fiber diet for a healthy digestive system.

In the 1930's, American doctors Cowgill, Anderson, and Dimmock supported the studies of those British doctors, promoting high fiber diets as wonderful aids in keeping digestive disorders at bay.

In post-World War II years, three physicians delved further into the "Fiber Hypothesis." Dr. T.L. Cleave, Dr. Hugh Trowell, and Dr. A. Walker did studies in the British Isles and in Third World countries, comparing digestive ailments in Great Britain to those in India and Africa. They found that the digestive illnesses common in Great Britain were almost non-existent in the less those countries. One thing found in Third World diets that was missing in diets in the modern countries was high fiber. Those countries had refined and processed all of the roughage out of their food, and, as a result, they suffered from digestive diseases that ranged from constipation to ulcerative colitis, stomach ulcers, and colorectal cancer.

A High Fiber Diet Is Very Difficult To Maintain!

It seems with all of this scientific information showing the need for high fiber to combat digestive disease, it would be easy to correct our errors by simply eating better. Unfortunately, this involves a commitment to diet change that most of us would find daunting. We would have to replace the foods which contain ultrarefined flours and sugars with whole grains; eliminate fried foods and those containing animal fat and tropical oils; and eat many more raw vegetables and fruits. This might read more easily than it actually is. Look at the ingredients of the foods stored in your pantry and refrigerator, and you will see how difficult it might be.

An Easy Source Of High Fiber!

Now that we know the need for diet change, but also face the dilemma of how to supply it, what is the answer? The best way to add high fiber to our diets without having to drastically change our lifestyles is by taking dietary fiber supplements.

A Stressful, Busy Life Can Cause Digestive Problems And Ulcers!

In this hectic, fast paced society, pressures of job, family, finances, and a multitude of other stressors often manifest themselves in physical ways in our bodies. When the pressures become too great, our bodies break down. Two common, interconnected signs our bodies show when stressed are digestive problems and stomach ulcers. If we haven't had these problems ourselves yet, we probably know someone who has. Do you have a friend who, when in a stressful situation, reaches into his or her pocket or bag, takes out a familiar brown prescription bottle and pops a few tiny pills into their mouth? A look of relief may shortly follow this gesture.

The Tagamet Alternative—
Another Answer For Ulcer Sufferers!

What your friend has most likely just done is take the prescription drug TAGAMET. A recent study shows that, over the last three years, doctors in the United States have prescribed more than $3 billion worth of the drug to ulcer sufferers. TAGAMET is very effective.

Unfortunately, it also has some side effects. One of the most disturbing for men taking the drug is gynomastia, or breast enlargement. According to TAGAMET'S manufacturers, only 4% of the drugs users encounter this problem, and they feel that the percentage is so small that there should be no concern. Of course, if you were among those affected, it would be very disturbing, and you would want an alternative treatment.

What doctors most often do not tell ulcer sufferers is that there are other options to TAGAMET that are both non-prescription, and that produce no similar side effects. One such treatment is deglycyrrhizinated licorice root (DGL). Doctors may tell you that licorice root does have side effects, like headaches and high blood pressure, especially when taken in large doses. Plain licorice root does contain a component called glycyrrhizinic acid, which can cause these side effects. Fortunately, with DGL, scientists have found a way to remove 97% of the glycyrrhizinic acid and still keep the excellent antiulcerative properties.

DGL Works Differently!

While TAGAMET and other prescription ulcer drugs work by decreasing acid secretion in the stomach, DGL aids your intestines and stomach in producing protective mucus. In the case of ulcer patients who must take aspirin, cortisone, or anti inflammatory drugs (which can produce or promote ulcer), this extra production of protective mucus can be extremely beneficial. It should be noted that scientific studies have proven that DGL tablets perform better in the treatment and maintenance of ulcers if they are chewed before swallowing.

A Germ May Be The Cause Of Chronic Stomach Irritation And Ulcers!

Although stress can play a large part in promoting ulcers or digestive problems, such as chronic stomach irritation (gastritis), scientists have very recently been linking these digestive disorders to the growth in the digestive tract of a germ called *Helicobacter pylori*. Researchers say, that our chances of being infected with the germ increases by 1% with each year that we live. In other words, by the time we're 50, we will have a 50% chance of being infected with *H. pylori*.

A Simple Test Can Tell You If You Are Infected!

Luckily, there is a simple test, that has proven 100% accurate, called enzyme-linked immunosorbent assay (ELISA). It can be done in your doctor's office, and in seven minutes you will know if you have *H. pylori*. Once this is determined, a treatment of antibiotics and Pepto Bismol can eliminate it. Tests of ulcer patients have shown that the treatment seems to heal ulcers permanently. Research physicians are also studying the possibility of using vitamin C and beta-carotene to kill the bacteria.

Almost Everyone Has Had Some Kind Of Digestive Distress In Their Lifetime!

Even if ulcers do not plague you, it is probable that some form of digestive distress has touched you. How often have you reached for that little roll of antacids, or mixed up that bubbling concoction to help soothe your aching stomach and calm your "heartburn"? Although they can be effective, these over the counter antacids can hardly be called natural.

A natural digestive aid is available called bromelain. It is an extract of pineapple juice, that has been used for centuries to help in soothing indigestion. Bromelain is quite safe and shows no known side effects.

Sources of Substances Mentioned
In This Chapter:

Most of the products discussed in this chapter are available at health food and vitamin stores. In addition, the following is a list of mail or phone order suppliers:

Bromelain:
Vitamin Research Products
2044 Old Middlefield Way
Mountain View, CA 94043
1-800-877-2447
or
The Vitamin Shoppe
4700 Westside Avenue
North Bergen, NJ 07047
1-800-223-1216

DGL:
Enzymatic Therapy, Inc.
P.O. Box 1508, 510 Lombardi Avenue
Green Bay, WI 54305
or
The Vitamin Shoppe
4700 Westside Avenue
North Bergen, NJ 07047
1-800-223-1216

19

Diabetes Problems Can Be Reduced And Even Eliminated!

Although diabetes is thought to be caused by various hereditary, physiologic and dietary factors, its true cause remains unclear. In most cases, it is characterized by persistent hyperglycemia (high blood sugar) and decreased glucose (sugar) tolerance.

Diabetes is classified into various categories. Type I diabetes requires daily injections of insulin a hormone normally secreted by the pancreas when blood sugar levels are increased, such as after eating. Type II diabetes may or may not require insulin, and can sometimes be treated with other medications.

Diabetes can sometimes develop during pregnancy, but usually resolved after delivery. Certain drugs, including some blood pressure medications, hormones, and medications that treat various psychiatric disorders, can also create this condition. Dietary patterns sometimes play a role as well.

Symptoms Of Diabetes!

The common symptoms of diabetes are frequent urination, excessive thirst and hunger, blurred vision and rapid weight loss. The onset is usually quite sudden in children and more gradual in adults. The diagnosis is confirmed by obtaining a blood sample after fasting for several hours and measuring the glucose level.

Different Treatment Options!

Left untreated, diabetes can cause damage to the arteries and nervous system, as well as metabolic abnormalities. Fortunately, there are numerous ways to treat this condition. Along with various types of insulin, there are medications in tablet form that can lower blood sugar. In mild cases, diabetes can sometimes be controlled by diet, combined with weight loss when appropriate.

Benefits From Plants!

In addition, research aimed at natural treatments for diabetes has yielded promising results. In Ayurvedic medicine, which has been practiced in India for centuries, extracts of the *Gymnema sylvestre* plant have been found to lower blood sugar, cholesterol and triglycerides to normal levels.

The *Journal of Ethnopharmacy* also reported that the benefits of the Gymnema plant extract "apparently resulted from the repair and/or regeneration of the actual insulin-producing cells of the pancreas." These results were observed in adults as well as in children.

Flax Oil—Not Just For Diabetes!

Another substance that has been successful in diabetes control is flax oil, which is a potent source of omega-3. Although a low-fat diet is recommended for everyone, including diabetics, the omega-3 contained in flax oil has been shown to increase the body's response to insulin. A study documented in the *New England Journal of Medicine* revealed that omega-3 fats "...were the most effective in overcoming very profound whole-body insulin resistance." Additional benefits of omega-3 oil are lowered cholesterol and triglycerides, as well as a strengthened immune system.

Surprising Benefits From Minerals!

Vanadyl sulfate is derived from the element vanadium. In animal studies, comparatively large doses of vanadyl sulfate resulted in almost normal blood sugar levels. Although the therapeutic dosage for humans has not been established, it is thought to be in the range of 20-75 mg after meals. Vanadyl sulfate is available without prescription.

Other minerals are helpful in controlling blood sugar. Chromium encourages production of GTF (glucose tolerance factor). GTF contains chromium, niacin and amino acids, and is required for normal glucose metabolism.

Magnesium deficiencies are common in diabetics, and supplements are thought to help prevent the eye problems that frequently accompany diabetes.

Decreased potassium levels are associated with elevated blood glucose and impaired insulin response, and are often present in obese patients. Increased potassium intake improves the body's use of glucose and increases insulin production.

Vitamins That Help!

Besides being part of the glucose tolerance factor, studies have shown that niacin increases glucose metabolism in smaller doses (50 to 150 mg). Vitamin B_6 alleviates peripheral neuropathy, a side effect of diabetes that damages the nerves in the extremities.

Diabetics who need insulin injections frequently have decreased levels of vitamin B_{12} and can develop anemia. Research studies have found that B_{12} supplements can improve diabetic retinopathy, another possible side effect of diabetes that affects the vascular systems of the eyes. Thiamine deficiencies are also found in Type I diabetes.

Diabetes can be managed with careful attention to diet, weight and proper medication. In some instances, improved eating habits, weight loss and exercise can reduce or even eliminate the need for insulin or other medication. However, it is important to work with your physician to monitor blood sugar levels frequently. Although natural therapies have been shown to help in diabetes control, please follow your doctor's advice before changing or discontinuing any prescribed treatments.

All of the supplements discussed in this chapter are readily available in health food and vitamin stores. Two additional sources of *Gymnema sylvestre* are Natrol, Incorporated, 20371 Prairie Street, Suite 7, Chatsworth, California 91311, and the Vitamin Shoppe, (800) 223-1216

icines

ruses from contaminated food,
blood transfusions. It becomes
nto the bloodstream that produce

t deposits from too much alcohol,
ious to cell regeneration, causing
is unable to process and filter the

ed, our body's chemical treatment

ure Liver Disease!

iver disease, a long list of scientific
inese and many European cultures
re's a botanical garden of protecting
natural affinity to the liver.

es act like blood brothers in prevent-
some, like *Taraxacum officinale*, aka
ackyard.

ooth-like leaves are rich in vitamins,
catalytic substances that help the liver

s that aid in cell metabolism, dande-
f bile in the liver and gallstones and

alleviates bile duct inflammation,
Dr. D.B. Mowery in the *Scientific*

If it becomes infected through v
syringes, needles, sexual secretions, an
inflamed and enlarged, releasing toxins
fever, fatigue and yellow jaundice.

If the liver becomes damaged by f
then its hardened cells become imperv
scarring or cirrhosis of the liver. Then i
blood.

In short, if it's not properly treat
plant becomes it's own toxic waste site.

Dandelions Help Cu

Working against the ravages of l
studies have confirmed what the Ch
have recognized for centuries–that the
compounds and substances that have a

These compounds and substanc
ing and alleviating liver disease. And
the dandelion, are right in your own b

This plant's seeds, stems and t
minerals, protein, pectins and other
purify the blood of toxins.

Containing enzyme-like agent
lions also stimulate the secretion
gallbladder surgery.

As a result, the dandelior
hepatitis, and jaundice, as repo
Validation of Herbal Medicine

Contains More Vitamin A Than Carrots!

Other studies show that the dandelion has anti-inflammatory proper-ties and protects against liver enlargement. Dr. H. Santillo in *Natural Healing With Herbs,* confirms that dandelions have a high mineral content, which helps cure anemia.

The *Encyclopedia of Common Natural Ingredients Used in Food, Drugs and Cosmetics* reports that dandelions contain more vitamin A than carrots, explaining its therapeutic value in curing a variety of liver disor-ders.

Choline Helps Remove Fat!

Additionally, dandelions contain the chemical choline, which plays a catalytic role in the breakup of fatty acid deposits in choline produced a fatty liver similar to alcohol-induced fatty liver in humans.

And while choline has not been shown to have a lipotropic or fat removing effect in treating this condition in humans, it has a remarkable affinity to another amino acid that does–methionine.

Methionine Is A Boozer's Best Buddy!

This catalytic compound is the liver's best protection against alcohol induced fatty liver. Methionine is a sulfur containing amino acid that stim-ulates the body's production of lipotropic or fat removing agents and helps metabolize fatty acids, according to Dr. R. Montgomery in "Biochemistry: A Case Oriented Approach."

Methionine also guards against the depletion of glutathione in the body which is essential to the metabolism of alcohol.

Glutathione is a sulfur-containing protein that combines with toxic agents like alcohol and converts them into water soluble compounds that are then eliminated from the body by way of the kidneys.

By restoring high levels of glutathione to sustain this metabolic process, methionine has become the weapon of choice in defending the liver against alcohol induced liver damage.

The Amazing Milk Thistle Plant!

Extracts from the milk thistle plant have profound effects on treating all types of liver disease, from acute viral hepatitis to cirrhosis.

The fruit, seeds and leaves of this plant, a member of the daisy family, contain the principle substance silymarin, which is more potent than vitamin E, as reported by Dr. R.F. Weiss in *Herbal Medicine*.

Silymarin, a flavonol, helps prevent liver tissue damage by scavenging free radical agents that are the offspring of fatty acid metabolism, according to Dr. H. Hikino in the journal *Planta Medica*.

Dr. Hikino also found that silymarin stimulates the liver to synthesize its own chemical scavengers which ingest these toxic particles and eliminate them from the system.

No Side Effects!

Its therapeutic effects have been confirmed by a wide range of studies, which showed that silymarin protects against such damaging chemicals as carbon tetrachloride in animals. It's also safe and doesn't contain debilitating side effects of some liver drugs.

Good News For Fat Lovers And Drinkers!

What's more, silymarin even helps synthesize proteins in the liver that produce new liver cells to replace damaged old ones, according to Dr. H. Wagner in *Natural Products as Medicinal Agents*.

Like methionine, silymarin also prevents the depletion of glutathione, offering drinkers double protection against alcohol induced fatty liver.

That's good news for people who like to drink and want to protect themselves against alcohol related liver diseases.

It's also good news for people who like to eat and are reluctant to give up high fat, low fiber diets that contribute to fat buildup in the liver.

Carnitine To The Rescue!

Carnitine is another substance that causes the breakup of these fatty acid villains. Manufactured in our own bodies, this vitamin like compound facilitates the conversion of fatty acids into energy, neutralizing their damaging effects on the liver.

A 1984 study by Dr. D.S. Sachan appearing in the *American Journal of Clinical Nutrition* suggests that alcohol impairs the body's ability to synthesize carnitine and, thus, its ability to convert fatty acids into energy.

Dr. Sachan asserts that higher levels of carnitine in the body are necessary to handle the toxic overload from alcohol and high fat diets. By supplementing the liver with carnitine, those levels are restored, preventing fatty acid deposits from building up in the liver.

Several Botanicals Also Help!

Extracts from the plant, *Cynara scolymum*, have an impressive track record in treating liver disorders. The active ingredient, cynarin, aids in the excretion of cholesterol and also stimulates the liver's ability to regenerate cells, according to Dr. H. Wagner in "*Plant Flavonoids in Medicine.*"

The Gallbladder Supplements
The Liver's Bile System!

With over 20 million Americans diagnosed with gallstones' attributed from high fat/low fiber diets and alcohol, maintaining the livers ability to manufacture and transport bile is crucial.

Another plant, *Curcuma longa*, helps stimulate bile flow. Because of this ability it is specifically prescribed for gallbladder disorders in preventing the formation of gallstones, according to Dr. A.Y. Leung.

Artemisia capillaris and *Canna indica* are two more botanicals that help stimulate bile flow. Additionally, *Canna indica* also protects the liver against viral hepatitis.

As reported by Dr. H.M. Chang in *Pharmacology and Application of Chinese Materia Medica* virtually 100 out of 100 cases of viral hepatitis were cured with mixtures of *Canna indica,* which made symptoms disappear.

Hepatitis: You're Always At Risk!

While millions of Americans are courting this disease through indiscriminate sex and contaminated needles, millions more are unintentionally exposing themselves through contaminated food.

Public health officials in Colorado recently reported an outbreak of hepatitis among 30 school children who became infected when a food server negligently failed to wash his hands. Barely escaping an epidemic, the conclusion is obvious. Everyone is at risk.

Prevents Yellow Jaundice!

Like uninvited guests at a party, eliminating viral hepatitis from the system isn't easy. But a number of investigative studies have confirmed that many natural substances have a profound therapeutic effect in treating the disease.

Uncaria Gambier, also known as catechin, is a flavonoid that significantly reduced serum bilirubin levels in patients suffering from acute viral hepatitis. The increased presence of bilirubin toxins in the blood lead to jaundice, a sickly pale yellowing of the skin.

In a double blind study reported by Dr. H. Suzuki in the medical journal *Liver*, catechin improved liver blood tests twice as fast than in the control group.

In another double blind study, the control group experienced a return of appetite and more rapidly overcame symptoms of nausea, weakness, stomach pain, and jaundice with skin color returning to normal in a short period of time.

Angelica Sinensis Inhibits Viral Reproduction!

Angelic sinesis (gentian root) is another natural substance shown to inhibit viral reproduction in 40 cases studied. It also improves immune system functions and increases red blood cell count and is effective in treating anemia.

The gentian root is effective in treating jaundice. Clinical studies, according to Dr. H.M. Chang, revealed that it had healing effects on 27 out of 32 patients suffering from hepatitis.

Extracts of the plant, *Glycyrrhiza glabra*, is yet another in the long line of natural substances that inhibit viral reproduction in chronic hepatitis, according to Dr. Suzuki. It's also been shown to protect the liver against damage from toxic chemicals.

Vitamin C Promotes Liver Health!

The beneficial role of vitamin C in promoting liver health has been well documented in several studies. Dr. F. R. Klenner, in the *Journal of Applied Nutrition* confirmed that daily doses of 40 to 100 grams of vitamin C, administered to patients with viral hepatitis, significantly relieved symptoms in two to four days and cleared up jaundice within six days.

A double blind study concluded that two grams or more of vitamin C each day prevented all participants in a controlled group of hospitalized patients from developing hepatitis B.

Other studies report that vitamin C protects the liver from tissue damage by helping eliminate free radical agents formed after the metabolic breakdown of fatty acids.

Protecting Your Liver
May Lengthen Your Life!

Longevity, say nutritional experts, is directly related to the health of your liver. In a toxic waste environment where exposure to liver damaging agents has never been greater, scientists emphasize the importance of liver protectant therapies to insure longer, healthier lives.

"Considering that there are 600,000 tons of pesticides and herbicides dumped into the environment each year," states Dr. Jane Heimlich, a noted nutritional authority. "We had best learn how to support the liver, or it will just swell up and leave us very, very sick."

Preventive Care Beats 911!

If you're a drinker and want to protect against fatty acid deposits which could lead to cirrhosis, Dr. Heimlich recommends a liver detoxification program two or three times a year that calls for taking 200 to 250 milligrams of silymarin daily for a month.

If you currently have a liver problem, she recommends six weeks of therapy with daily doses of silymarin. For people who want to give up alcohol, specialists recommend two grams daily of l-glutamine, which lessens the craving for alcohol. Additionally, one gram per day of l-carnitine helps improve fatty acid metabolism.

Better At Night!

There are studies that indicate when you drink is more important than how much, states Dr. John D. Palmer of the University of Massachusetts, who reported that liver metabolism is slower between noon and 2 P.M. and burns 25% faster in the early evening. In other works, three vodka tonics at night beats a dry martini at lunch.

For non-drinkers exposed to chemicals and pesticides, doctors recommend a formulation of liver protectors that can combat these damaging agents.

Sources Of Substances Mentioned In This Chapter:

Most of the products mentioned are available at health food and vitamin stores. You might also locate some in Chinese herb shops.

Taraxacum officinale (dandelion root)
Choline
Methionine
Silymarin (milk thistle)
Carnitine
Cynarin
Artemisia capillaris
Silymarin
Canna indica
Catechin (Uncaria Gambier)
Angelica sinensis, (gentian root)
Glycyrrhiza glabra
Vitamin C
Curcuma Longa

Mail-order sources for these substances are available through:

Ethical Nutrients (800-692-9400) and L & H Vitamins (800-221-1152).

A product called D-Tox contains many of these substances, such as: carnitine, silymarin, cynarin, methionine, *Artemisia*, liver extract, *Taraxacum*, *Angelica* and glutathione. D-Tox is available from:

Gero Vita International,
Dept. Z101,
2255-B Queen Street East #820,
Toronto, Ontario M4E 1G3, Canada,
(800) 825-8482

21

Hair Loss May Be Reversed–And Not With Rogaine (Minoxidil)!

Picture in your mind a man in his late, late 40's nearing that landmark of "middle age"–the turn of a half century of living,

You probably will envision such a 50-year-old showing some bare scalp at the top of his head. Male pattern baldness is a common phenomenon. Also there are many women who have concerns about thinning hair as well, if not actual bald areas on their scalps.

Lifestyle And Hair Loss!

Can elements within our lifestyles play a role in helping accelerating or decelerating hair growth? Dietary deficiencies can contribute to gradual hair thinning. Serious disorders of the endocrine glands, such as the thyroid or pituitary, can result in hair loss. Exposure to nuclear radiation or the anticancer drugs are well known for the unfortunate baldness they produce as a common side effect.

Inherit The Bald Spot?

Baldness is an inherited trait that is found with higher frequency among males. It's that male hormone, testosterone, which is the culprit here. In fact, hormonal imbalance may in part produce early baldness.

It is well known that a more sudden type of baldness can be produced by stress factors. Sometimes hair will turn gray almost overnight. Other times it will actually fall out. Illnesses such as the flu, typhoid fever or pneumonia—even excessive stress—all can play a role in helping create that shiny bald spot.

The Best Elixir Of All
Or Side-Effect Hell?

There is one pharmaceutical drug on the market which has been shown to produce hair in balding men. After all the hullabaloo, the problem with ROGAINE is that you have to keep using it forever! Stop the Rogaine and hair growth stops. Even worse, the hair that had been growing in falls out! Besides the relatively high cost factor, it has been found to be more effective on younger men who have male pattern baldness but only recently began to lose some of their hair.

Another unfortunate aspect of Rogaine is that sometimes it produces hair where the recipient might prefer it not appear! So you better be careful where you apply it.

Natural History Of Hair Follicles!

The life of each hair on your head has a beginning and an end. But contrary to popular belief, hair growth is not continuous. If allowed to grow without being cut, a hair might reach three feet in length. That strand could sit on your head for three, four or even five years! Perhaps that would lead one to have the impression that hair growth is continuous.

There are three phases of hair growth. The anagen phase is when the hair is growing actively. With the proper release of energy, hair is generated and develops well in the right environment. For example, a chemical compound, PDG, is known to stimulate hair production. Dr. D. Adachi, in 1987 at the World Congress of Dermatology, discussed the mechanism of this hair growth compound which is called in scientific circles, glucose "6" phosphate dehydrogenase, or PDG.

When hair growth slows down, it enters the catagen phase. During this period, there is a tapering of the growth pattern, until the hair stops growing altogether and eventually falls off the scalp. The latter represents the telogen phase. Obviously if we could shorten the catagen and prevent the telogen phases and keep the anagen phase going, there would be many fewer scalps showing!

Keep That Hair Normal!

Under normal conditions, 90% of the hair found on a person's head is in the andogen phase. Only 10%, therefore, has stopped growing or will be falling off in the shower or onto the hairbrush and comb. If one could help the hair follicle switch back into the andogen phase, then perhaps hair loss could be prevented!

In the June 1990 issue of the *Journal of Anti-Aging Breakthroughs*, Dr. Kugler writes that "using the same type of sophisticated biological assay techniques as have produced new miracle antibiotics, scientists began prying into the cell's energy mechanisms. They knew from previous research that DHT (dihydrotestosterone) could block a key energy reaction, so that is where their first suspicion fell."

This provided the path for hundreds of researchers around the world to begin to research those substances which could cause a switch of hair follicles out of the catagen or telogen phases and back into the andogen phase.

Where did the path lead to? "Odd numbered fatty acids," wrote Dr. Kugler. "After evaluations of almost three hundred different materials,

Japanese researchers led by Dr. Kenkichi Oba demonstrated that application of a high energy-related substance found in actively growing hair, such as 3-carbon compound of pentadecanoic acid glyceride caused a 350% increase in the production of ATP in animal tests."

Give It The Right Energy And
Hair Will Grow!

Dr. Oba has written about different products that stimulate hair growth. Helping the energy level during the anagen phase can prolong hair growth, he points out. Apparently, where baldness sets in, there is a reduction in the energy metabolism in the follicle.

Dr. Oba has shown that PDG (the same as G6PHD) even outperforms Rogaine. It seems to increase the metabolism of the hair roots and counteracts the androgenic hormone which hails the anagen or falling off the skull phase. Using PDG with 253 volunteers, men ranging in age from 27 to 62, were then evaluated by 19 dermatologists in a double-blind clinical test. The PDG solution won over the falling hairs! Both men and women can take comfort in knowing it is permanent help.

Dr. Oba did not observe any harsh side effects in blood analyses, liver functions or in urine samples. Now PDG has a big following in Japan and Germany.

Perhaps the best known nutrient for healthy hair is biotin. This coenzyme assists carboxylation reactions (introducing carbon dioxide into a compound with resultant formation of carboxylic acid). In the case of the follicular energy cycle, empirical data have been gathered that show its power to renew hair growth when applied topically. This process can reverse the pattern involved in balding—thinning and depigmentation of the hair.

Other Stimulants For Natural Hair Growth:

Ginseng roots have been used medicinally for thousands of years in China. Dr. John Chang reported in *Cosmetics and Toiletries Magazine* on the use of ginseng for prevention of loss of hair. Apparently it offers protection to hair and prevents brittleness.

It has been found that it is possible to extract and refinel hinokitiol oil from a Japanese tree, called hiba. Also a similar oil from the western red cedar can be extracted as well. The result is (b-Thujaplicin), which was discovered in Formosa by Dr. Zozao. Hinokitiol has a very rare seven membered organic ring compound, or carbocyclic chemical.

When hinokitiol copper salt was mixed as an ingredient in a tonic and used to treat areas deprived of hair, Japanese studies showed that thicker hair growth occurred. Then, at the University of Nihon's Department of Dermatology, a study was done with 11 patients, both male and female. Downy hair growth occurred between seven and 60 days.

Another study using hinokitiol was conducted at Chiba University's Department of Dermatology. This time 10 patients were treated for alopecia areata. Here, 60% effectiveness was noted, with downy hair growing within two months. Another study performed in a Tokyo hospital on 50 patients yielded similar results (68% effective in growing downy hair).

Still More Anti Balding Agents!

Other remedies include Orizanol, a derivative from rice oil, which stimulates microcirculation and acts as an antioxidant. Also there is a Japanese botanical that is applied topically to stimulate hair roots to hasten growth, called swertia (toyaku in China).

Another Japanese product, Takanal, demonstrated in a clinical study 92% effectiveness in growing downy and, eventually, coarser hair. It has been approved for use in cosmetic preparations by the Japanese Ministry of Health and Welfare.

In one study published by Dr. Takashima in the 1985 *Journal of Clinical Therapeutics and Medicine*, a placental extract was used on the scalps of 27 balding men. Over 70% were noted to have a reduction in hair loss. The explanation was that the placental extract was a kind of cell enhancer or activator. The application of the extract led to additional oxygen being provided to the cells from the blood; hence, hair rejuvenation.

Three Amino Acids Promote Hair Growth!

There are three amino acids that are known to offer nutritional support to hair. These are cysteine, serine and glutamic acid. Dr. Nishimjima, from Japan, added Takanol to the amino compound that he applied topically to the scalp. In his work, the addition of Takanol brought an ample supply of these amino acids which are not easily available through diet, and the result was accelerated, thicker hair growth.

There are trichopeptides (amino acids directly affecting the hair) which stimulate the receptors that enhance cell growth. Dr. Mendes and Dr. Taub, two scientists from Europe, tested 60 people with trichopeptides, both men and women, who suffered from alopecia. They were successful in the majority of cases and noted that the women had a 100% improvement!

Tri-Genesis Proven In Tests!

Double blind tests show that a compound called Tri-Genesis produced a 227% increase of vellus hair count within six months.

AMA Laboratories, an independent certified testing laboratory in New York, performed a clinical study using the standard double blind methods over a six month period of time. Dr. Martin Schulman directed this study of Tri-Genesis, which was reviewed by a board certified dermatologist.

In addition to the remarkable increase in hair count, this study showed that 78% of the people studied had a successful outcome. More than three quarters of the subjects who participated in this study benefited with improved hair growth. Clearly, such success might be worth investigating before resorting to more drastic procedures such as surgery.

Dr. Hans Kugler, scientist and author of *Slowing Down The Aging Process* and editor of the clinical journal *PreventiveMedicine*, discovered the key ingredient that is now used in the Tri-Genesis formula.

This essential component of the product is naturally occurring source of a unique, uneven-chained (odd-numbered) fatty acid, *a-angelica lactone*. It has been found that this ingredient dramatically reduces the resting stage of air follicles and actually gives each hair a tremendous burst of energy.

Paves The Path To Baldness Prevention!

The Japanese confirmed the results of Kugler's test. Dr. Oba discovered what a specific odd-numbered fatty acid was doing to cause hair growth. *Science Forum 2000*, reported, "His team found biological evidence how uneven-chained fatty acids increased the amount of ATP (energy) to the hair follicles. In 1987, governments in Japan and Germany approved the sale of products containing these active agents."

Another scientist, this time from China, developed an herbal formula to prevent hair loss. When the skeptical Japanese examined Dr. Zhao's formula, they found safflower extract, ginko and ginseng, all excellent vasodilators.

Rogaine Is A Vasodilator

The action of a vasodilator is to enhance blood flow. In the case of hair, when there is a more abundant supply of blood to the hair follicles, this nourishment seems to enhance hair growth. Perhaps this explains why so many people have hair loss, including those who often lose hair prematurely. They may not be receiving ample blood supply to the roots of their hair.

A fourth herb Dr. Zhao used was angelica, a type of aconitum. Remember Dr. Kugler's key ingredient, a "unique uneven-chained odd-numbered fatty acid, *a-angelica lactone*?" The essential ingredient in Tri-Genesis is angelica.

All Useful Nutrients Are In One Product!

The Tri-Genesis formula contains many of those substances which have been found to be effective in hair growth stimulation. The innovative contribution by those who created this product, however, is that the various active ingredients can now all be found within the same formula. To summarize, these ingredients are:

TRF or Tissue Respiratory Factors in liposomal delivery system helps cells use oxygen. The critical phase of oxygen uptake, before the anagen phase, is when these factors come into play which is just before the changes occur that result in enhanced hair growth.

B-Glycyrrhetinic acid, also in the liposomal delivery system, acts as an anti-inflammatory agent and is a reductase (a enzyme) inhibitor.

Biotin is a coenzyme for carboxylation reactions (introduction of oxygen) in the follicular energy cycle. Topical application has resulted in rejuvenated hair.

Oleum serenoa repens liosterolic is an extract which counteracts the conversion of testosterone to dihydrostestosterone (DHT) and inhibits DHT binding to cellular and nuclear receptor sites, thereby increasing DHT breakdown.

Swertia is a source of 5-hydroxygenteopicroside (Swertianmarin), and has been shown to activate ATP, DNA and G6PDH activity.

Danggui extract is a source of 15-hydrdoxypentacecanoic acid which has shown to increase follicle ATP, DNA and G6PDH activity.

Pregnenolone acetate exercises dermatographic activity similar to B-estradiol with no hormonal side effects.

A-Angelical actone derived from 15-hydroxypentadecanoic acid, increases follicular metabolism.

Sodium undecylenate-NA, (salt of undecylenic acid) is a fatty acid which occurs in sweat and may contribute to increased follicular metabolism.

Undecylenamid DEA, an undecylenic acid diethanolamide, has anti-fungal and anti-dandruff activity.

Tocopheryl acetate enzymatically bioconverts in the skin into an active form which activates ATP, DNA and G6PDH in hair follicles.

Tocopheryl nicotinate improves blood flow.

Niacin improves blood flow and accelerates function.

Conclusion!

As you have seen, a major breakthrough has been achieved in the area of male pattern baldness. Even given the inherited trait, it may be possible to stimulate those follicles not to give up and keep on growing. Just give them what they need.

Sources Of Substances Mentioned In This Chapter:

A number of the products mentioned in this chapter can be located in health food and vitamin stores in your community such as biotin, ginseng root and swertia.

Further information about Tri-Genesis is available by writing to Tri-Genesis Corp., 520 Washington Boulevard, Suite 385, Marina del Rey, California 90291; or call 1-800-654-0456.

Products such as hinokitiol, Orizanol and Takanal MIGHT be found in Japanese or Chinese pharmacies or herb shops in the major cities in the country.

There are herbal preparations which can be found in local health food stores that will contain one or more of the ingredients listed in this chapter, although not necessarily specifically prepared for purposes of hair regeneration. Check with your local merchant.

22

Stop Insomnia, Jet Lag, Breast Cancer And Live Longer!

Melatonin is a hormone secreted by the pineal gland located in the brain. It is produced during periods of darkness. Until recently, its role in human health was not well understood. However, numerous worldwide studies have now revealed varying uses for melatonin which may have wide-ranging benefits.

Melatonin Helps At Bedtime!

Sleep patterns vary from person to person, and are affected by such factors as age, chronic pain, breathing problems, or emotional disturbances like anxiety or depression.

As people age, they require less sleep. Although this change may be described as insomnia, it is a normal phenomenon and can be managed by increasing exercise during the day and using various relaxation techniques. When sleeplessness often stems from anxiety, it is usually temporary and is resolved as the troublesome situation is solved. Breathing problems such as sleep apnea can be treated with surgery, weight loss or medication.

Although various medications are prescribed in some cases of insomnia, prolonged use is associated with the risk of addiction, overdose, and increased tolerance, which leads to the need for higher doses in order to fall asleep. In addition, sleep patterns can be disturbed once the drugs are discontinued, creating in a cycle of dependency. This also results in confusion, anxiety and symptoms of dementia, especially in the elderly.

Sleep Without Side Effects!

Therefore, sleep experts discourage long-term use of sedative medication and recommend natural methods to induce sleep once other causes of insomnia are ruled out. Melatonin has been quite effective in this regard and in very low doses has been found to aid sleep.

Since the pineal gland receives information from the optic nerves, darkness signals melatonin production to increase. Very little is released in daylight. As melatonin levels rise in the bloodstream, a sedative effect is obtained, thus inducing sleep. In cases of insomnia, a natural substance such as melatonin would be ideal, since it is non-addictive and allows deep sleep, unlike more conventional sleep medications.

A study in the journal *Biologic Psychiatry* demonstrated that when persons with insomnia took melatonin before bedtime, they slept for longer periods, without impairing their daytime alertness. Additional research described in *Psychopharmacology* indicated that melatonin helped patients fall asleep faster, stay asleep longer, and they had heightened energy levels upon awakening.

Dr. Al Lewy, of the Oregon Health Sciences University in Portland, has conducted numerous successful experiments with low doses of melatonin, enabling adults to shift their body clocks forward and backward. Dr. Lewy believes that these findings can be applied to those who must work varying shifts, so that they can adjust to their changing schedules more easily and avoid the health problems caused by lack of sleep.

Valerian—Nature's Sedative!

Another natural sedative is valerian, which has been used for centuries. As Dr. Olov Lindahl reported in a study published in *Pharmacology, Biochemistry and Behavior*, "Valerian has been used as a medication for as long as historical information has been available."

Dr. Peter Leathwood conducted a study of valerian which was also documented in *Pharmacology, Biochemistry and Behavior*. The one hundred and sixty-six subjects who participated reported improved sleep after taking valerian capsules, without the usual "hangover" feeling associated with conventional sleep medications. In addition, smokers in the study found that they slept more soundly.

Valerian is non-addictive and its effects are not amplified by alcohol intake, thus eliminating two of the risks of narcotic sleep medications. As Dr. Andrew Weill noted in his book *Natural Health, Natural Medicine*, "Valerian is a safe and effective sleeping aid, more powerful than l-tryptophan or such sedative herbs as hops and skullcap." In addition, it provides relief from such stress-related symptoms as headache, irritability and fatigue. Valerian is commonly used in Europe. In France, for example, over one million people take valerian capsules regularly.

Recover From Jet Lag Quickly!

Crossing multiple time zones in a short period of time is a fact of life for many people today. However, air travel can cause a phenomenon known as circadian dysrhythmia, or "jet lag."

Characterized by fatigue, disturbed sleep patterns, impaired concentration and various other symptoms, jet lag usually requires twenty-four to forty-eight hours before the body adjusts to local time. It is also thought that the effects of jet lag can be diminished by gradually adjusting sleep patterns to the destination time a few days before departure, eating a high-protein, low-calorie diet and avoiding alcohol while in flight.

In addition to its ability to safely induce sleep, melatonin has also been found to alleviate the symptoms of jet lag in travelers.

A double-blind study published in the *British Journal of Medicine* reported on ten male and female subjects of varying ages who were given 5 mg of melatonin before, during and after a round-trip flight between London, England and Auckland, New Zealand. When compared to the group that was given a placebo, those who received melatonin resumed their normal sleep patterns more readily and had increased energy.

Possible Breast Cancer Prevention!

Researchers are examining many factors to explain the increased incidence of breast cancer, including aging, diet, heredity, hormonal influences, and radiation. Improved diagnostic techniques are finding more cases earlier, which may also influence the statistics in this area.

Once diagnosed, breast cancer can be treated with conservative or radical surgery, radiation, anti-cancer drugs, or a combination of these therapies. Although they can be successful in halting the spread of the disease, all of these treatments have varying risks and side effects.

Melatonin has shown potential benefit in breast cancer treatment. In laboratory tests, breast cancer cells exposed to melatonin did not proliferate (grow). A study from *In Vitro Cell Developmental Biology* revealed that melatonin slowed tumor growth.

A similar finding was also noted by Dr. Randy Nelson of Johns Hopkins University in Baltimore. After placing laboratory mice in summer and winter light conditions, they were given carcinogenic (cancer-causing) substances. None of the mice who lived in the darker, winter light conditions developed cancer, while 85% of the mice exposed to summer lighting did. Since melatonin is produced in darkness, it was considered to be the protective factor in this study.

The drug tamoxifen, which has also shown promising results in breast cancer treatment, was found to be one hundred times more effective on patients who first received melatonin, according to an article in the *Journal of Clinical Endocrinology and Metabolism*.

Interestingly, it has also been observed that Japanese women, who have a comparatively low incidence of breast cancer, have higher levels of melatonin than women from other countries. Melatonin is commonly found in certain seaweeds which are used for food in Japan.

Slow The Aging Process!

In addition to its other properties, melatonin has also shown the potential to delay the aging process. At the Institute of Integrative Bio-Medical Research in Switzerland, Dr. Walter Pierpaoli noted that mice lived for the equivalent of twenty additional human years when given melatonin, and that many symptoms related to aging were delayed or even reversed.

As Dr. Keith Kelley reported in *Medical Hypotheses*, "Melatonin deficiency syndrome is perhaps the basic mechanism through which aging changes can be explained in a simple causative action. This may require replacement of melatonin in order to achieve a more youthful endocrine balance...and subsequently repair the body as a whole."

Decreased levels of melatonin are thought to adversely affect all body systems, causing them to operate less efficiently and creating changes commonly associated with aging. 25-year-olds have four times the level of melatonin in their bodies as 60-year-olds. As a result, Dr. Pierpaoli suggests that daily melatonin supplements be taken daily after age 60, and believes that by doing so, 90 to 100-year lifespans are possible.

Additional Benefits Of Melatonin!

Melatonin has also been found to lower cholesterol, according to Dr. Georges Maestroni of the Institute of Pathology in Locarno, Switzerland.

In his study, subjects with elevated cholesterol who were given melatonin experienced a 15-30% decrease in LDL (artery-clogging) cholesterol, while those with normal cholesterol levels were not affected.

In addition to its positive results in breast cancer treatment, melatonin supplements may also help men diagnosed with prostate cancer. In a study documented in the *Journal of Neural Transmission*, Dr. H. Bartsch noted a relationship between decreased levels of melatonin and the development of prostate cancer.

Seasonal affective disorder (SAD) is a form of depression that occurs in some people during the winter months when there is less daylight. By treating this condition with exposure to bright light during the day, it is believed that increased melatonin production results during the night, thus lessening or eliminating depressive symptoms.

Undoubtedly, future research will reveal new uses for melatonin, and its role in maintaining health will be further clarified. For now, adequate sleep each night is the best way to insure adequate melatonin levels in the body.

Sources Of Substances Mentioned In This Chapter:

Valerian is available in many health food and vitamin stores. Melatonin may also be found in some stores. If it is not available in your area, call: Life Extension Foundation, 1-800-841-5433 or 305-966-4866.

Sleep Aid made from valerian root is available from: Gero Vita International, Dept. Z101, 2255-B Queen Street East #820, Toronto, Ontario M4E 1G3, Canada, or call (800) 825-8482.

23

You Can Live Longer, Healthier, No Matter How Old You Are Now!

Until recently, medical science has been more concerned with the treatment of diseases associated with old age than with aging. Scientists have only seriously begun to look at the causes of aging in the last decade.

In the United States in 1900 the average life expectancy for a man was 49.5 years; in 1955 the average rose to 68.5 years. Today the average life span in America is about 72.1 years for the males and 79 years for females, a 46% increase since the turn of the century!

Dr. K. G. Kinsella, in an article for the *Journal of Clinical Nutrition*, credited the increase in life expectancy to "...Expansion of public health services and facilities, combined with disease eradication programs to greatly reduce death rates, particularly among infants and children."

You Have A 25% Chance
Of Becoming A Centenarian!

The *Wall Street Journal* reported that in 1950 the probability of a 65 year old American reaching age 90 was 7%, but 40 years later it is 25%. According to *USA Today*, in the past decade the number of Americans 100 years or older doubled to 35,800. The *Wall Street Journal* predicted that by 2050 the number of centenarians would number in the millions.

After the age of maturity, usually around 25 to 30 years, the body begins to deteriorate at the rate of .7% a year. The average weight for an adult human brain is 1,500 grams. At the age of seventy, the brain's mass is reduced to 1,000 grams. One third of the brain is no longer there! Along with the brain, every major organ in the body is affected by this slow-process. This self destruction process has been confirmed by Dr. Roy Walford, one of the nation's leading anti-aging researchers and founder of the immunological theory of aging.

Improved Quality Of Life For
The Elderly Is On The Horizon!

Although serious research on the aging process is fairly new, there have been a number of discoveries that not only promise to raise the maximum life span, but the quality of life will be immeasurably increased as we grow older!

"What drives most of this research is not the desire to be immortal, it's the desire not to die in a nursing home," says Dr. Richard Sprotta, biologist with the National Institute of Aging. "I think most of us would trade dying at age 85 rather than 105 if we knew we could be healthy up to 85, then we could have one last cigar or bourbon and kick off."

How Scientists Are Manipulating The Genes That Control Aging And What To Expect In The Future.

Dr. Michael West, a molecular biologist at the University of Texas Southwestern Medical Center in Dallas, discovered that two mortality genes, M-1 and M-2, can speed aging or reverse the aging process, depending on whether they are turned "on" or "off". In an experiment reported in the *Chicago Tribune*, Dr. West successfully turned the M-1 gene "off". Aging cells normally have the M-1 turned in the "on" position. The aging cells reversed their aging, becoming younger and increasing the number of times they could divide. By turning the M-2 gene off, cells appeared to go on agelessly, dividing indefinitely.

Dr. West told *Chicago Tribune* reporters, "There is no turning back, for the first time in history we have the power to manipulate aging on a very profound level." He went on to speculate that by controlling these genes, life expectancy would eventually extend to 200, 400 or even 500 years.

Dr. Michael R. Rose, at the University of California at Irvine, has successfully bred a strain of fruit fly that is able to live twice as long as ordinary fruit flies. The super flies are also far more robust than their ordinary counterparts. They produce a more effective form of the cellular antioxidant, superoxide dismutase. Dr. Rose told *Scientific American*, "The work on drosophila is trial run stuff for doing the same thing in mice. If we can create long-lived mice, specific genes, enzymes and cell processes involved in longevity should be revealed."

Science Doubles Lifespan In Tests!

Dr. Thomas Johnson, a biologist with the Institute for Behavioral Genetics at the University of Colorado in Boulder, discovered that the life span of roundworms can be doubled by altering one gene. This was the first successful attempt to significantly increase an animal's life span through manipulation of genetic controls. *Scientific American* reported,

"Strikingly, the mutant worms produce elevated levels of antioxidants (both cytoplasmic superoxide dismutase and an enzyme called catalase) and are more resistant to the toxic effects of paraquat, a herbicide that leads to generation of the superoxide radical."

Based on research by molecular biologist Dr. Thomas Maciag of the American Red Cross's Jerome Holland Laboratory for the Biosciences, it was discovered that the life span of skin cells is doubled by switching off a gene that controls production of the protein called interlukin 1. The technique used by Maciag to turn off the gene is called antisense. Antisense is currently used to create ageless tomatoes that stay ripe indefinitely.

Researchers Find Key To Immortality!

Dr. Judith Campisi, of the Lawrence Berkeley Laboratory, discovered that shutting off the gene c-fos stops the gene's fibroblasts from duplicating their DNA. This prevents cells from dividing, and the aging process continues. However, after using a special substance to turn c-fos on, the cell's reproductive process continues, and aging stops.

Dr. W. Wright and Dr. J. Shay, from the University of Texas Medical Center, have found a genetic mechanism that causes cells to die. The researchers discovered a way to deactivate this "death" mechanism. Cells with the deactivated mechanism live indefinitely without aging.

Human Life Span Not Set In Stone!

Dr. Richard Cutler of the National Institute on Aging Gerontology Research Center in Baltimore says that the human life span is not set in stone. He sees no reason why our descendants won't achieve an average life expectancy of 200 years.

Free Radical Causes Aging!

There are theories–other than the genetic cause of aging–that are receiving attention from prominent scientists the world over. The free radical theory of aging has received the most attention and positive results achieved through antioxidant treatments are proven without a doubt. The free radical theory of aging is based on importance of oxygen. Dr. Denham Harmon is considered the founder of the Free Radical Theory of Aging. Beginning in 1954, he formed one of the most important theories on life extension developed in the twentieth century. Harmon asserts that oxygen based compounds (oxygen free radicals) in the human body are primary causes of aging. "Chances are 99 percent that free radicals are the basis of aging," says Harman.

In an article written for the *Chicago Tribune*, Dr. R. Kotulak amplified, "Aging is the ever increasing accumulation of changes caused or contributed to by free radicals."

Dr. Earl Stadman, chief of laboratory of biochemistry of the National Heart, Lung and Blood Institute in Bethesda, Maryland, agrees that damage from oxygen free radicals contributes heavily to accelerating the aging process. The free radical theory is more important than science was previously willing to accept. Life span is dependent on cellular damage caused by oxygen free radicals. The body's cells do resist some oxygen damage, but eventually these cells become so damaged that they can no longer function.

Studies suggest that oxygen free radical reactions cause the age related deterioration of the cardiovascular and central nervous systems. Dr. Harmon says that free radical reactions may also be significantly involved in the formation of the neurotic plaques associated with senile dementia of the Alzheimer type. Senile people showed higher levels of plaques than those found in normal people.

Free Radicals Compared To
The Great White Shark!

Time Magazine describes free radicals as "...great white sharks in the biochemical sea. Cellular renegades wreaking havoc by damaging DNA, altering biochemical compounds, corroding cell membranes and killing cells outright, scientists believe such molecular mayhem plays a major role in the development of ailments like cancer, heart or lung disease, and cataracts. The cumulative effects of free radicals also underlie the gradual deterioration that is the hallmark of aging in all individuals."

Oxygen free radicals differ from other molecules in the fact that the electronically charged particles (electrons) that make up free radicals are unpaired and unbalanced. The chemical process for creating energy in the human body is an imperfect process. It often strips an electron from an oxygen atom, creating an unpaired electron and a very unstable molecule. This alone sets the free radical apart. Their action against cells is called oxidation.

Did you ever notice metal rusting or an apple turning brown? These are common examples that we see occurring everyday caused by the process of oxidation. Eventually the metal and the apple will slowly disintegrate to nothing.

Free Radicals Believed To Be The Cause Of Many Diseases!

Free radicals are elusive and extremely difficult to study, as they live only a millionth of a second. Yet many respected scientists believe that oxygen free radicals are responsible for numerous ailments affecting the human body. These illnesses include; atherosclerosis, Alzheimer's Disease, cancer, Parkinson's Disease, Down's Syndrome, stroke, paralysis, cataracts, arthritis, emphysema, wrinkling, memory loss, and the list is increasing daily.

The free radical needs a matching electron from another molecule and searches frantically for a mate. This process of searching causes cellular mayhem. The free radical molecule clashes with other molecules in an effort to attract an electron. The constant assault by free radicals on other molecules destabilizes molecules within other cells. Once generated, they grab on to everything they reach. And once triggered, free radical reactions tend to be unstoppable, uncontrollable, and irreversible, almost explosive.

Free Radicals Speed Formation
Of Brown Spots On Skin!

Free radicals damage the body in a number of ways. By damaging fatty compounds, it causes them to turn rancid, which in turn generates the release of more free radicals. Free radicals are responsible for the loss of the optimal function of cellular membranes, which disrupts nutrient absorption and waste disposal, and ultimately, causes the death of the cell.

Throughout its short life span, one free radical can damage a million or more molecules. "Free radicals alter cell membranes in such a way as to kill the cell or change it into a cancer cell. Free radicals can also bind compounds together in such a way as to alter their function or the physical characteristics of the entire tissue. As an example, young baby like skin can be made tough as leather by the actions of free radicals produced by sunlight," reports Dr. Passwater, author of *The New Supernutrition*.

Free Radicals Cause Wrinkles!

It is believed that free radicals damage the coded message of genes and damage enzymes in its search for an electron. Dr. Roy Walford, one of the nation's leading anti-aging researchers, is convinced that cellular processes that occur in the mitochondria are also affected.

Oxygen free radicals destroy the proteins that are essential elements of our body. Protein regulates hormones and enzymes that make up the various nerves, muscles, skin and hair. Damaged proteins cause one of the more obvious signs of aging—wrinkles.

DNA Affected By Free Radical Damage!

Free radicals also damage DNA. It is thought that many substances that cause or promote cancer may do so by stimulating cells to produce free radicals, which damage or alter the cell's blueprint until the cell becomes cancerous.

Free radicals promote cross linking between DNA and protein, which prevents DNA from carrying out its replicative duties, and instead produces cellular garbage. DNA is the hereditary blueprint for life within each cell and is responsible for the orderly reproduction of cells. If one strand of DNA is damaged, reproduction of the cell may be adversely impacted. Damaged DNA may cause birth defects, cancer and other diseases, as well as decreased production of the proteins that make up the essential elements of both enzymes and hormones.

Combating Free Radicals
Key To Slowing Aging!

Dr. Bruce Ames, director of the National Institute of Environmental Health Sciences at the University of California at Berkeley, estimates that the genetic materials in each cell are hit 10,000 times a day by free radicals.

Free radicals are chemical terrorists. The key to slowing aging, preventing cancer, heart disease, and arthritis, along with protecting the body from other ailments, is to reduce the number of free radicals.

Dr. Harmon and Dr. Hans Kluger claim that researchers have three avenues that must dictate future research. The optimum level of naturally occurring antioxidants must be established; new and improved antioxidants must be discovered; and the best combination of antioxidants must be determined for optimum effectiveness.

Free Radical Fighters!

It follows that if there is one basic cause of aging, and if the damage caused by oxygen free radicals can be confined, aging can be controlled. Dr. Harmon's research in studies involving animal subjects demonstrated that their life spans correlated with their ability to repair free radical damage. He maintains that our bodies have the ability to control free radical damage before they inflict too much harm.

In 1981 Dr. Harmon recommended that future diets should contain "...increased amounts of substances capable of decreasing free radical reaction damage, such as a-tocopherol (vitamin E), absorbic acid, selenium or one or more synthetic antioxidants." Studies have shown that when these substances, which are designed to counter the effect of free radicals, are added to diets of experimental animals, average and maximum life span increases do occur.

For example, even though the human body produces its own antioxidants, the materials needed for optimal antioxidant production are not always present in the required quantities in the food we consume. Materials such as zinc, copper and manganese are required by the body to manufacture super oxide dimutase (SOD), one of the body's most important free radical fighters.

Antioxidants, Nemesis Of Free Radicals!

"Nature has developed within each cell the ability to manufacture protective free radical neutralizers, or to use the more popular term– antioxidants," says Dr. Walford.

In a report published in the *Journal of Medical Sciences*, Dr. Harmon states that animal subjects, who were given antioxidants in a double blind study, had virtually no tumors when they died, compared to the control subjects who had many. Studies indicate that antioxidants such as ethoxyquin, a chemical feed additive, and 2-mercaptoethylyne (MEA) have increased life spans significantly.

Dr. Harmon notes that the addition of MEA, an antioxidant first developed by the Atomic Energy Commission to protect against radiation exposure, to the diets of experimental mice, "...increased life span by 30 percent." This increase is equivalent to raising the human life span from 72 to 95. MEA's strength as an antioxidant is particularly effective in preventing damage caused by iron based, oxygen free radical compounds.

Iron Based Free Radical Compounds Are Dangerous!

A provocative study by Finnish researchers, published in the American Heart Association's scientific journal, Circulation, concluded that the amount of iron stored in the body ranks second only to smoking as the strongest risk factor for heart disease and heart attacks.

US News & World Report, cited experts in placing iron ahead of high cholesterol, high blood pressure and diabetes as a leading cause of heart attacks.

Dr. Hans Kruger, Ph.D., explained, "Your body produces hydrogen peroxide as a byproduct of metabolism, the burning of oxygen. Scientists believe that iron combines with hydrogen peroxide in the body to cause a cascade of cellular-damaging oxygen free radicals that can damage heart muscles as well as the nerves and fatty acids of the heart.

Damage of these nerves may mean that you will need a pacemaker in your later years to renew electrical nerve impulses to the heart that can no longer be efficiently transmitted from your brain. Furthermore, oxygen free damage of your heart's circulatory tissues can mean that you may need heart surgery—if a heart attack doesn't strike first!

Vitamin E Is More Important To The Heart Than Cholesterol Damage!

Although vitamin E is one of the most commonly found antioxidants, it is not to be underestimated in its free radical scavenging ability. Dr. Harmon asserts, "The declining death rate from gastric carcinoma in the United States may be related to the introduction of breakfast cereal, particularly wheat cereals, rich in tocopherol (vitamin E) and other antioxidants."

In research performed in 16 European cities for the World Health Organization, it was discovered that men with the lowest level of vitamin

E in their blood were more likely to suffer fatal heart attacks than those with the highest levels. The link was so obvious, cholesterol levels were ruled out as a factor between those with the lowest and highest levels of the antioxidant in their bodies.

According to Dr. Daniel Steinberg of the University of California in San Diego, there is a "...reasonable amount of evidence..." showing antioxidant supplements like vitamin E actually help prevent arterial disease.

Dr. Robert Bolla. of the Roche Institute of Molecular Biology, reported in the medical journal, *Archives of Biochemistry* that the antioxidant tocopherol increased life span by 19% in experimental animal subjects.

PBN Declared Effective In Restoring Memory Loss!

Dr. Robert Floyd, a molecular toxicologist at the Oklahoma Medical Research Foundation, and Dr. John Garvey, of the University of Kentucky, have used the antioxidant PBN with surprising results. The researchers demonstrated that memory loss caused by free radical damage can be restored in aged animals! Aged gerbils were given PBN for two weeks to stop free radical damaging processes. The gerbils were forced to use their memories in order to escape physically confusing enclosures. The PBN treated older gerbils performed as well as the younger, untreated gerbils.

Memory Loss Can Be Overcome!

Floyd and Garvey's results with the PBN treated gerbils prompted Dr. Earl Stadman, chief of the laboratory for biochemistry of the National Heart, Lung and Blood Institute in Bethesda, Maryland, to declare that age related memory loss could finally be overcome by reversing oxygen free radical related cellular damage.

U.S. Issues First Patent For Anti-Aging Pill, ACF223!

Dr. Richard Lippman, member of the New York Academy of Sciences, the Royal Institute of Technology and the Swedish Medical Association, developed the first patented anti-aging pill. The ACF223 formula consists of a combination of butylated hydroxytolene (BHT) with catalase, MEA , nordihydroguairetic acid (NDGA), vitamin E and citrus. When taken orally, ACF223 revitalizes the collagen and elastin fibers of the skin. It also chelates "free" iron and protects the heart from free iron consumed in foods.

It was discovered that one of ACF223's components, NDGA, enabled animals who inhabited the extremely hot deserts to withstand extreme ultraviolet radiation from the sun. The animals derived NDGA from eating certain cactus plants. Patients given one of the ingredients of ACF223 during experiments at Sweden's Department of Medical Cell Biology were reported to have a dramatic increase of blood oxygenation. Appearance, overall health, vigor and sex drive in the patients were significantly improved. Dr. Lippman said, "Conservatively speaking, antioxidant therapy has been estimated to slow the aging process at a mean rate of 15 to 20%."

Common Food Preservative Doubles As Free Radical Fighter!

Another component of ACF223, BHT, is one of the most common food preservatives in use today. It is known to be extremely effective in neutralizing oxygen free radicals and has been shown to be effective in preventing acute lethality in X rays, and prevents cancer causing chemicals from creating tumors.

NASA Tested Anti-Oxidants!

The antioxidant, TCA, clearly has an anti-tumor effect, says Dr. Brugarolis. He also reported that aged animals treated with anti-oxidants mate more often and act younger. At NASA's Ames Research Center, Dr. Jaime Miguel found that TCA increased life spans by 8 to 14 percent.

Earlier in the chapter, we discussed Dr. West's research on two mortality genes M-1 and M-2, and how they can be turned "on" or "off." These anti-aging genetic structures are referred to as Methuselah genes and they are responsible for the production of SOD, a powerful antioxidant.

Dr. Irwin Fridovich, Duke University biochemist, headed a research team that first discovered the existence of the oxygen free radical, super oxide, and its antioxidant cousin, (SOD). The discovery of SOD actually confirms that the body not only produces oxygen free radicals, but antioxidants as well.

The Missing Link?

One in three Americans will suffer from cancer, and about 22% of the population will die from this disease. Dr. Larry Oberly, one of the nation's leading SOD researchers, says, "Cancer is a disease that has resisted man's efforts at understanding since the beginning of its study. This lack of understanding is obviously because a vital link in the biochemistry of the cancer cell has been missing. Many groups around the world are now examining whether superoxide dismutase is that missing link."

Dr. Richard Cutler, of the Gerontology Research Center of the National Institute of Health in Baltimore, says that researchers have experimented with SOD's life extending properties on 12 species of mammals and found that those with the highest levels of SOD lived the longest.

Will SOD Lead Scientists
To A Cure For Cancer?

Studies of SOD in cancerous cells reveal that the levels of the antioxidant are greatly diminished at the time of malignancy. Dr. Oberly says, "If oxygen radicals are the cause of normal cell damage, and if low antioxidant levels in target tissue are potentiating factors, then these facts suggest that adding back antioxidants should prevent normal tissue damage."

Dr. Passwater notes that research has uncovered additional characteristics of SOD which enables the antioxidant to protect cells from various forms of radiation, including UV rays emitted by the sun, pollution from above ground nuclear testing, nuclear reactors and nuclear waste.

Lives In Nuclear Reactor!

Nuclear radiation creates free radicals, and it would be difficult to imagine anything surviving, never mind thriving at the core of a nuclear reactor. Yet, the bacterium, radiodurans, is able to survive the high radiation levels found in the reactor and seems quite content living there. Radiourans has more SOD per gram of body weight in its system than any other living organism on earth.

Researchers at Duke University's Department of Medicine and Biochemistry, using in vitro techniques (meaning studies performed outside the body), exposed one set of white blood cells to SOD and left the other set unprotected. Both sets of white blood cells were exposed to free radicals. The white cells containing SOD remained alive, the other set died.

A similar experiment was conducted at the Institute of Biology, Physics, and Chemistry in Paris, and the outcome was the same. Researchers added SOD to one culture and left the other culture alone in an in vitro study. Known carcinogens were added to both cultures. The SOD protected culture remained healthy and the other culture developed cancer.

Dr. Michael Rose, a biologist with the University of California, discovered that delaying reproduction in animals ultimately extended the life spans of future generations by as much as 80%. Dr. Rose concluded that the longevity of the test animals could be attributed to the selective breeding process. These selective animal strains possessed unusually high levels of SOD in their systems.

"Aging is associated with an increasing biochemical imbalance. Whether this is a cause or effect of the aging process is unclear. Most likely it is both, meaning that age changes may be partly the results of cells not having correct amounts of vital substances needed for their function," noted Dr. R. Hochschild in *Experimental Gerontology*.

Our Lives Depend On Our White Blood Cells!

Are we making sure that our white cells are in optimum fighting form? Scientists have determined that four substances which provide the ideal nourishment for our white blood cells. Alkylglycerols and N-Dimethyglycine (DMG) are the main ones. Phycoten and Echinacae, are plant substances that also nourish these cells.

Dr. Astrid Brohult became frustrated watching her young patients die from the dreaded cancer-leukemia (lack of white blood cells). Dr. Brohult assumed that white blood cells were created in the bone marrow. She cut into the bone marrow of a calf's leg and transplanted the marrow into one of her terminally ill patients. The transplant seemed to help, creating greater energy and increased blood cells.

Astrid's husband, Dr. Sven Brohult, promised his wife that he would analyze the marrow to see what had stimulated the production. Dr. Brohult spent years attempting to isolate the agent. Finally, he discovered that alkylglycerols were responsible for increasing the production of all types of blood cells. Alkylglycerol has a long chain of carbon molecules which play a major role in creating a certain white blood cell known as a "leukocyte".

Sharks Don't Get Cancer!

Unfortunately, known sources of alkylglycerols were extremely rare until scientists stumbled onto a Chinese secret. Chinese medicine prescribed shark oil to cure a number of ailments, from burns and cuts to increasing fertility.

It has been known for some time that sharks are the only animals that never develop cancer. Researchers subsequently discovered that liver oil from the Greenland shark contained approximately 30% alkylglycerols.

Alkylglycerols derived from sharks have been shown to limit or even arrest the growth of tumors. Dr. Cederberg reported success in increasing the white blood cells and platelet count in a number of AIDS patients.

Dr. Brohult found that alkylglycerols proved effective in alleviating both leukopenia (white blood cell reduction) and thromboctopenia (blood platelet reduction) in leukemia patients.

Patent Issued For DMG!

The U.S. Government issued a patent in 1986 for a substance called N-dimethyglycine (DMG), a synthetic version of alkylglycerol's second element. Based on glycine, the simplest amino acid in our bodies, DMG has the ability to increase human immune defense. This medium chain of molecules plays an important role in the building of antibodies. Dr. Elizabeth Reap says, "DMG has no known undesirable side effects."

Reduction In MAO Nets
A 21.2% Increase LifeSpan!

Dr. Ana Aslan, Romania's first female physician, cardiologist and the chief doctor for the Geriatric Institute of Romania, learned from the *Journal of Physiology* that there was an enzyme in our bodies called monoamine oxidase (MAO). The *Journal* reported that the level of MAO stays at about the same level until our mid-thirties, then increases dramatically as we grow older. People suffering from debilitating diseases such as arthritis, neuritis, arteriosclerosis, senility and depression were found to have much higher levels of MAO than the norm.

Using 920 aged white rats, Dr. Aslan conducted a series of experiments to see if she could lower MAO levels using various formulas. Dr.

Aslan discovered a combination which lowered the rats' MAO by 85% within a two week time frame. The rats with lowered levels of MAO lived 21.2% longer than normal.

Dr. Aslan used her formula on a patient who had been admitted to the hospital with arthritis so severe he could not move his leg. After agreeing to volunteer for the experimental treatment, the man found he could move his leg within a day after Dr. Aslan began the treatment. Two days later the man was released. He walked out of the hospital as if he never had arthritis!

A 109 Year Old Rejuvenated Using Dr. Aslan's Treatment!

Later, police brought a homeless, elderly man to the hospital. The dirty and disheveled cripple suffered from depression and loss of memory. He could not speak, and was in a terminal age of senility. Within a year, Dr. Aslan's treatment rejuvenated and restored much of the old man's lost or eroded functions. He was vigorous, alert, very mobile with much of his memory restored.

The publicity surrounding Dr. Aslan's success with the old man attracted the attention of a woman who recognized the rejuvenated man as her father. The woman brought in documents verifying the old man's true age as 109 years. He was an Armenian named Parsh Margosian.

Dr. Aslan's formula was named Gerovital H3 and primarily contains procaine, which is often used as an anesthetic.

111 Patients Lived 29 Percent Longer With Gerovital H3!

Over the next fifteen years, Dr. Aslan kept meticulous records on 111 patients who were taking her treatment. On the average, the test group lived approximately 29 percent longer than the average life expectancy.

Throughout the years, thousands of Dr. Aslan's patients reported improved or alleviated problems connected with aging, such as arthritis, neuritis, impotence, mental deterioration, memory loss, psoriasis, asthma, angina pectoris, ulcers, arteriosclerosis, depression, bad skin and muscle tone, no sexual drive, loss of energy, osteoporosis, and hearing loss. Some patients' hair also darkened.

Politicians And Movie Stars Rush To Romania For Treatment!

Dr. Aslan's research did not go unnoticed by the scientific community or high profile patients. Nikita Kruschev, Cary Grant, Kirk Douglas, Onassis, Marlene Dietrich, Prince Ranier, Somerset Maugham, Charles De Gaulle, Sukarno, Imeldo and Ferdinand Marcos, Stalin, and Chairman Mao benefited from Dr. Aslan's treatment.

Science Confirms Value Of Gerovital!

Dr. Joseph P. Hrachovac of the University of California (USC) found that Dr. Aslan's formula, Gerovital H3, reduced the monoamine oxide MAO level in the body by as much as 87%. Dr. David MacFarlane of USC confirmed Dr. Hrachovac's research.

Dr. Arnold Abrams of the Chicago Medical School performed double blind tests of GH3 that resulted in very positive findings. Based on these results, the enthusiastic Dr. Abrams visited Romania in order to obtain more information.

East German physician Dr. Fritz Wiederman treated over 600 patients with Gerovital H3 and remarked that "The results were stunning and happened very fast". To illustrate his findings, he gave reporters a file on a 67 year old female subject who was experiencing frequent bouts of crying. The woman also suffered from arthritis and a total inability to work. After undergoing treatment with Gerovital H3 for only one week, the woman was able to return to work.

Less than three months after beginning the treatment, her swollen hands were restored to their former size, and her arthritis pains disappeared. After five months, her hair regained its former color and began to grow in where it had fallen out. The most surprising result of the treatment was that, in her sixty-eighth year, the woman's wisdom teeth appeared, "...proving how extensive regeneration had occurred in her case," Dr. Wiederman remarked.

89% Suffer Less Depression!

In a report to the Gerontological Society, Dr. Keith Ditman, medical director of Vista Hill Psychiatric Foundation in San Diego and Dr. Sidney Cohen, professor of Psychiatry at UCLA stated that they found 89% of aging patients suffered less depression after taking Gerovital H3. Doctors Cohen and Ditman reported that the majority of patients who took the drug "...felt a greater sense of well being and relaxation, slept better at night, obtained relief from depression and the discomforts of chronic inflammation or degeneration disease."

At the annual meeting of the American Geriatrics Society in 1975, Dr. William Zung, professor of psychiatry at Duke University, and associate professor Dr. H.S. Wang, reported that their double blind test with Gerovital H3 and a placebo, showed significant improvement of mental condition of those getting Gerovital H3. Dr. Leonard Cramor, of the New York Medical College, conducted his own double blind test and later concurred with the findings of Dr. Zung and Dr. Wang.

Dr. Albert Semord, a prestigious member of the American Medical Association, the New York County Medical Society, the American Geriatrics Society and the New York Academy of Sciences, tested Gerovital H3 on 50 patients and himself for several months. He said, "Every month I'm more stupefied with the results–not only physically, but mentally and emotionally."

Gerovital Improves Sex Drive!

Dr. Semord said, "All my patients feel the same as I do. I don't look my age (78). I fish, I hunt, I ski. I make love twice a week. I feel extremely well." He reported that Gerovital H3 had "...an astonishing effect on his patients' mental clarity and emotional stability."

A number of MAO inhibitors are being marketed in the United States as antidepressants. Gerovital H3 proved to be a better inhibitor of MAO than prescription drugs, which produced liver damage, hypertension, chest pain and headache as side effects. Gerovital has demonstrated no side effects.

The main ingredient of Gerovital H3 is procaine. Dr. Pelton compares procaine to a computer that enables the body to "...return to normal whatever is abnormal, each milligram representing 240 millivolts of electricity."

Dr. Hochschild says, "By its very nature, this substance cannot be compared with any other...it neither stimulates or depresses in its many actions, but rather regulates and normalizes." Dr. Aslan concurred, "If you are tense, it will relax you. If you are listless, it will revive you."

Dr. Aslan confirmed procaine's ability to correct problems of the circulatory system. Procaine has been found therapeutic for the heart, and the vascular system and is a natural vasodilator.

Procaine's Secret Unveiled!

Dr. Hans Kruger discovered that procaine breaks down in the body to paraaminobenzoic acid (PABA) and 2-dimethyl aminoethanol bitartrate (DMAE). DMAE and PABA are well known substances contained in minute amounts of foods we eat. Dr. Kugler reports, "In my own longevity studies on cancer prone mice at Roosevelt University in Chicago, we used procaine as one of the life extending factors. In two animal studies, we compared procaine to the DMAE/PABA mixture and found literally the same positive results for the DMAE/PABA mixture as for procaine itself."

Until recently, the only way a person could benefit from procaine was by injection in a doctor's office. American scientists have developed an improved version of Gerovital H3 that does not require a prescription. A combination of DMAE and PABA is now marketed as Gero Vita GH3.

"In experiments with animals, PABA has worked with pantothenic acid to restore gray hair to its natural color," noted Dr. Earl Mindell.

DMAE Increases Lifespans 30 To 40%!

Today DMAE is one of the most essential and nutrients available to people who desire increased longevity. Although concentrations are minute, the natural presence of DMAE in living organisms has been demonstrated.

Dr. R. Hochschild says, "Because of its essential role in membrane biosynthesis, the present results suggest that the aging process can be influenced by maintaining proper concentrations of DMAE."

DMAE is found most abundantly in those foods which the public tends to think of as "brain" foods, such as anchovies and sardines. DMAE has the remarkable ability to cross the blood-brain barrier. Subsequent experiments have shown that the nutrient is responsible for extending the life spans of animals by approximately 30 to 40%.

Dr. Murphy reported the results of double blind tests conducted while he studied DMAE under grants from Riker Laboratories, the U.S. Public Health Service Mental Health Institute, and Geschickter Fund for Medical Research. The findings, published in *Clinical Pharmacology and Therapeutics*, stated, "Of the psychological and subjective responses, the significant findings were an increase in muscle tone, better mental concentration, and changes in sleep habits which were; less sleep needed, sound sleep, and the absence of the customary period of inefficiency in the morning in the DMAE-treated group." The majority of the group reported favorable effects such as "improved mood," "relief of headaches," and "clearer thinking."

Dr. Ross Pelton noted, "Results from the use of DMAE have shown that it elevates mood, improves memory and learning, increases intelligence and extends life span."

DMAE Manages Learning And Behavior Disorders!

DMAE also demonstrated effectiveness in helping to manage the learning and behavior disorders of childhood. It has also been used successfully in the treatment of Huntington's chorea. Dr. Osvaldo reported in 1974 that, "An average of 500 mg daily in children and 1,000 mg daily in adults seems to be necessary for achieving clear cut therapeutic effects. The best clinical effects have been achieved after three months of treatment in children and there seems to be a minimum period of time for best effects."

Dr. E. Miller reported the results of DMAE therapy in 11 Parkinsonian patients with dyskinesia. After providing a dosage between 500 and 900 mg daily, dyskinesias were completely eliminated in eight patients and greatly improved in a ninth. The therapeutic response began 10 to 14 days after initiation of treatment.

In his book, *Mind Food and Smart Pills*, Dr. Ross Pelton mentions that the U.S. Food and Drug Administration (FDA) originally allowed DMAE to be marketed as a prescription drug and authorized Riker Laboratories to market it under the trade name Deaner. Later the FDA asked for an efficacy study. Due to the small market for Deaner at the time and the costs involved in conducting the study, Riker discontinued the product.

Growth Hormone Reverses 20 Years Of Aging!

The body's production of growth hormone slows when people reach their 30s. In about one third of the population, production virtually stops at around age 60.

Dr. Daniel Rudman, of the Medical College of Wisconsin at Chicago Medical School, published findings of a study of the human growth hormone (GH) in the *New England Journal of Medicine*. The study examined the effects of GH on 21 healthy men between 61 and 81 years old. "What we saw over six months was that several of the body composition changes (of aging) were reversed," said Dr. Rudman. "These represented the reversal of one or two decades of aging with regard to these factors."

Dr. Rudman's research demonstrated an ability in rebuilding muscle mass in the aged. Scientists are of the opinion that the benefits are more wide ranging and rejuvenating. GH treatment increased the men's lean body mass (muscle) by 9% and fat tissue decreased 14%. Their skin thickened by 7%.

Dr. Mary Lee Vance of the University of Virginia, in an accompanying editorial to the GH double blind study, commented that the work is "an important beginning."

DHEA Benefits Immune System, Raises Energy Levels!

In a recent study performed by Dr. Eugene Roberts of the Department of Neurobiochemistry for Beckman Research Institute of the City of Hope, Duarte, California, dehydroepiandrosterone (DHEA) has raised levels of energy, endurance, limb power, strength and agility in patients suffering from multiple sclerosis, a disease effecting the central nervous system. DHEA enhances the immune system, prevents cancer and has immeasurable influences throughout the human body.

Ginseng And Ginger!

For centuries, ginseng and ginger have been known as "anti-aging" herbs in China. People knew that ginseng could be used to calm nerves, heal ulcers, and increase potency. Western researchers have recently confirmed what the Chinese had known for thousands of years.

Current research has shown that ginseng helps strengthen the immune system. Dr. Tsung isolated the immunostimulating polysacchrides within the ginseng in 1986. Dr. Ruriko Haranaka discovered that ginseng has powerful antioxidant qualities. The saponins inherent in ginseng's makeup have proven to lower cholesterol levels.

The journal *Modern Research* states, "Ginseng does not appear to possess any specific, well defined pharmacological action, but rather exhibits a large number of different pharmacological activities, all of which contribute toward its total therapeutic effect."

Pineal And Thymus Glands Affect Aging!

The scientific community believes that the malfunction of the pineal and thymus glands contributes to the start of the aging process in the body. Failure of these two glands to function properly causes a decreased ability to handle stress and every organ in the body is affected, physical and mental abilities decrease, and a person's appearance degenerates.

Melatonin Treatments Reverse Age Related Debility And Disease!

Scientists have discovered that the pineal gland secretes a neurohormone called melatonin. According to the medical journal, Medical Hypotheses, "The Melatonin Deficiency Syndrome is perhaps the basic mechanism through which aging changes can be explained in a single causative action. This may require replacement of melatonin in order to achieve a more youthful endocrine balance, and consequently repair the body as a whole."

In a double blind study published in the journal *Immunology* by the Swiss Institute For Integrative Biomedical Research, it was reported that aged animals receiving melatonin live 20 percent longer: "Melatonin not only prolonged their life, reversed or delayed the age related debility and disease, but they were more youthful, bright, mobile, had better skin and hair quality and were more vigorous. Melatonin exerts profound influence in the regulation of our defense mechanisms."

In respect to the thymus gland, Dr. N. Fabris reported that, "Decline in thymic activity is not an irreversible event, and some nutritional intervention, such as amino acid treatment, may reactivate the production in the thymus. Recently, it has been shown that arginine accelerates wound healing and increases thymus weight. Some aspects of immunological decline with advancing age can be corrected with arginine and lysine (amino acids that stimulate growth hormone production)."

Chromium Picolinate Increases Life Span In Rats 36%!

The mineral chromium picolinate has made the news recently as a nutritional supplement that can prolong a person's life. Dr. Gary Evans, professor of chemistry at Bemidji State University in Minnesota, recently concluded a four year study on the effect of chromium picolinate on aging. Dr. Evans announced the results at the joint meeting of the American Aging Association and the American College of Clinical Gerontology at San Francisco in October of 1992. Rats receiving chromium picolinate had a median life span of 45 months, compared to 33 months for rats receiving other types of chromium. This represents a 36% increase in lifespan!

The Search For An Anti-Aging Solution Is Coming Of Age!

Advances made by science in recent years reflect the public's increasing demand for longer and improved life spans. This demand is also reflected in funding trends.

The federal government's National Institute of Aging is the fastest growing branch of the National Institute of Health, with a budget that nearly doubled from $222 million in 1989 to $402 million in three years later.

Now that scientists are receiving serious funding for anti-aging research, our quest to achieve what was once thought impossible is finally within our grasp.

Sources Of Substances Mentioned
In This Chapter:

The following are available in many health food or vitamin stores (If you don't find some of these on the shelves, the proprietor can order them for you): Alkylglycerol, arginine, BHT, catalase, copper, chromium picolinate, DMG, ginger, ginseng, PABA, vitamin E and zinc.

The Human Growth Hormone (GH) and Procaine are available by prescription only. TCA, PBN and MEA are available only to scientists for experimentation.

Gerovital H3 is only available in Europe, however the American version, Gero Vita GH3 which also contains PABA and DMAE is available from Gero Vita International, Dept. Z101, 2255-B Queen Street East #820, Toronto, Ontario M4E 1G3, Canada, or call (800) 825-8482. SOD is an ingredient in Super Shield, another product made by Gero Vita International. They distribute ACF223 which also may be found in a few vitamin and health food stores.

24

Healthiest Doctors Take Six Times The "RDA" Of Vitamins And Minerals— And So Should You!

These days, it seems almost everywhere you look—from the side of your box of breakfast cereal to television advertising for foods and patent medicines—you'll see boasts about nutritional content. All these listings and claims are designed to prey on our interest in maintaining good health and well-being through proper nutrition. But what do they mean in terms of the nutrients our bodies actually require for optimum health?

According to federal law, the nutritional content of food is given as a percentage of the Recommended Daily Allowance or RDA. This is the government's estimate of the MINIMUM amount of each nutrient the average person in good health requires each day to stay healthy. But as a guideline to our true nutritional needs, many nutritionists and researchers have concluded the RDA is a very poor yardstick for measuring how much of each nutrient you really need. If you get just the minimum RDA, you are on the borderline between sick and healthy.

Nutrition Does Affect Your Health!

Before the 1750s, sailors on long sea voyages frequently developed bleeding gums, wounds that refused to heal, rough skin, and muscles wasted, all symptoms that characterize the disease called scurvy. Back then, before refrigeration, sailors subsisted primarily on a diet of biscuits and dried meat, with very few fruits or vegetables. Thus, the stage was set for one of the first scientific experiments in nutrition.

A British Navy doctor divided the sailors aboard the fleet's ships into two groups. Both groups got the usual rations, but one group was also given limes to eat at sea. The group on the standard rations alone, as expected, continued to develop scurvy. But the group that got the limes—and in them the key nutrients we now know as vitamin C and bioflavonoids—avoided sickness.

The results of this experiment were too dramatic to ignore, and soon the order went out that all hands were to be given limes or other citrus fruits to eat on long voyages, which is why British sailors are known as "limeys" to this day.

In fact, the theory of a disease being caused by something lacking in the diet—a deficiency disease—was proven.

Sick Rats Determine The RDA!

Following the 250-year-old British Navy model, the United States government sponsors testing to determine how much of a nutrient we need to avoid developing a vitamin deficiency disease.

Using rats or mice on a controlled diet, a particular nutrient is eliminated until the animals become sick. Then the researchers gradually add small amounts of the nutrient being tested to the diet until obvious signs of deficiency disease disappear and the rats are able to reproduce. The amount is carefully measured.

Calculating the weight ratio between the average rat and the average human, and tacking on a small percentage to account for variation in adult human body size and the needs of pregnant women and lactating mothers, the government arrives at its Recommended Daily Allowance—that is, the absolute minimum amount your body requires to avoid getting a deficiency disease.

But is staying one step ahead of the ravages of deficiency disease the same thing as optimum health?

Vitamins And Minerals:
How Much Do You Really Need?

These were the questions that fascinated one of America's most brilliant scientific minds over thirty years ago as he set out to discover what level of nutrition is required to be truly healthy.

Dr. Emanuel Cheraskin, professor emeritus at the University of Alabama Medical School, is both a medical doctor (M.D.) and a dentist (D.M.D.). His curriculum vitae runs to well over 40 pages because he has written or co-written 23 books and has published over 700 scientific papers in prominent medical journals. Dr. Cheraskin has been honored worldwide for his significant medical research and has received 210 citations in the National Library of Medicine.

Dr. Cheraskin wrote, "America is 17th (of the countries of the world) in life expectancy at birth...(and) Medicare costs for the oldest (of our citizens) may increase sixfold by the year 2040." "It is unlikely," Dr. Cheraskin continued, "that these projected increases...will be restrained solely by cost containment strategies."

Instead of basing his work on calculating the level of malnutrition where rats would develop deficiency diseases in order to deduce human nutritional needs, Dr. Cheraskin took a completely different tack.

To Find Out About Health, Look At Healthy People!

Dr. Cheraskin reasoned that if a person was free of any symptoms of illness, such as aches, pains, colds, allergies, and abnormal functions such as high blood pressure, then they must be healthy. He decided to study a group of these very healthy, people to see what level of nutrition was contributing to keeping them that way. Being a doctor and a dentist, he didn't have to look far for his experimental group. Medical professionals became Cheraskin's subjects because they knew the importance of good nutrition and a healthy lifestyle. And, they could afford the best food and medical care.

For over 20 years Dr. Cheraskin surveyed, interviewed, and monitored 1405 dentists and their spouses.

To assemble this group, Cheraskin sent thousands of dentists across the country both the Cornell Medical Index Questionnaire and the Standard Food Frequency Questionnaire. The Medical Index asks for the mildest symptoms of ill health, even though actual sickness may not be present. The Food Questionnaire requests an inventory of what you eat, how much you eat, what supplements you take, and how much of each supplement you take.

Good Nutrition Promotes Good Health!

The initial survey of dentists revealed what Cheraskin suspected all along—that healthy people kept themselves well nourished both through diets and by taking supplemental vitamins and minerals. What he didn't expect to see was the dramatic correlation between nutrition and health: the lower the level of nutrition, the higher the incidence of symptoms of poor health—and, conversely, the higher the level of nutrition reported, the less frequent and less severe the symptoms.

For the next twenty years, Dr. Cheraskin conducted hundreds of double blind studies to scientifically confirm his survey findings of the direct relationship between good nutrition and good health. In these studies, half the subjects were given vitamin supplements and half were given placebos. No one except Dr. Cheraskin knew which participants got the real vitamins and which got the fakes.

Dr. Cheraskin methodically tested every vitamin, every dietary mineral, and every trace nutrient thought by science to be needed by human beings—and he tested some that remain controversial to this day. His goal: to establish, based on human testing, the ideal amount of each nutrient required daily for the "most healthy" life.

He proved that the optimally nourished body repairs itself more effectively, fights off germs better, and delays cell damage longer.

RDA Standards Demolished!

In all his studies, Dr. Cheraskin and his research team consistently found optimum nutrient levels to be FIVE TO NINE TIMES GREATER THAN THE GOVERNMENT'S RDA!

During all these years, the government did not significantly change its RDA levels, but Dr. Cheraskin's findings were gaining notice in the scientific community, and other scientists were conducting research of their own.

Cheraskin's Results Confirmed
By Independent Studies!

A study conducted for the Eli Lilly Company by Dr. Judy Z. Miller, for example, examined the effects of vitamin C on child development.

Dr. Miller studied identical twins six to 11 years old. One twin ate a normal diet, and the other ate the same diet but ALSO took a supplement of vitamin C five times the RDA amount. After only five months, amazing results were already obvious.

While the children on the normal diet grew at the expected rate, all but one of the children receiving the supplementary vitamin C grew faster, outstripping their identical siblings by 1/4" to more than a full inch!

In another experiment, Dr. W. A. Harris tested the effects of mega-doses of vitamin C on infertile men. Forty men were enrolled in the test. Half were given a gram of vitamin C every day for two months. The other half were given a placebo. In a truly sensational result, ALL of the wives of the men given the vitamin C became pregnant during the experiment, and NONE of the wives of the men taking the placebo conceived.

Perhaps our modern diet is seriously deficient in the level of nutrients needed for optimum health. But don't we eat better now than ever before? Dr. S.B. Eaton reported in the *New England Journal of Medicine* on his team's research into the nutrition of Paleolithic people. They found that the plant and fruit diet of our early ancestors gave them an average daily vitamin C intake of 392 mg (very similar to Dr. Cheraskin's ideal level of 349 mg)—and way above the RDA.

How Many Nutrients Are Really Important For Good Health?

Dr. Cheraskin's three decades of research revealed that there are some 30 VITAMINS, MINERALS, BIOFLAVONOIDS AND ENZYMES essential to good health—and most of them are needed in amounts far greater than specified by the government's RDA. For example, the healthy, symptom free people he studied had intakes of vitamin A five times greater than the RDA, intakes of vitamin B_1 nine time greater than the RDA, and consumed more than five times the RDA of vitamin C. And bioflavonoids and enzymes are not on the government list at all, even though research has demonstrated they are essential for good health!

Are You "Clinically Well"?
Only 5% Are!

Based on his studies, Dr. Cheraskin estimates that only about 5% of the adults in the United States would be rated very healthy, or, as he puts it, "clinically well" after answering the Cornell and Food Frequency questionnaires.

Our most obvious experience with disease is the sudden onset of an illness we catch, such as a cold or the flu. Few of us realize most illnesses are progressive in nature, beginning as a relatively slight imbalance or infection and progressing in severity over time unless the underlying cause is identified and treated.

Dr. Cheraskin theorized, that diabetics for example, gradually progress from being just slightly diabetic—say, 5%—until they are completely diabetic years later. In many cases recognizing the symptoms early can be the first step in reversing the progress of the disease before it is too late.

Even relatively minor health problems, according to Dr. Cheraskin's reasoning, can be an indication of a potentially serious health crisis down the road. With this in mind, he looked at his most "symptomless" subjects to help determine his model for what constitutes the nutrition you need for optimum health.

Good Health Habits
Can Help You Be "Symptomless"!

Along with proper nutrition, good health habits are essential for a long and healthy life. One of the best guidelines for developing a healthier lifestyle is a federally funded study conducted in Alameda County, California.

This 14 year plus study of hundreds of Alameda residents revealed that people who practice at least six of seven good health habits live an average of 11 years longer than those who practice fewer than two good health habits.

The good health recommendations studied were:

1. Get eight hours or more of sleep each night.
2. Maintain proper weight for height and bone structure.
3. Refrain from smoking.
4. Drink no more than two glasses of wine or one drink of hard liquor per day.
5. Exercise moderately three time a week.
6. Eat a healthy breakfast daily.
7. Eat meals during regular hours.

These results were confirmed by the nation's largest ever health research program, the decades long Framingham study of residents of the Boston suburb. In all, hundreds of well researched, well reported studies point to the conclusion that is possible to live longer and healthier by following simple good health habits, including eating a careful diet and taking nutritional supplements.

An Optimal Nutrition Program Can Make A Dramatic Difference In Your Health!

For years, we've been admonished to eat a sensible balanced diet. But just what constitutes a diet optimized to keep us as healthy as possible?

The outline of Dr. Cheraskin's optimal nutrition program is fairly simple, but it is quite different from the typical diet of most Americans. Included in his plan are elements designed to provide the nutrition needed to keep our bodies operating at peak efficiency while helping to ward off infections, minimize progressive conditions brought about by deficiencies and imbalances, and slow aging.

In the foods we eat, the Cheraskin plan considers our need for organic nutrients, including carbohydrates, proteins, lipids (fats, fatty acids, cholesterols) and vitamins. Organic nutrients are all compounds based on the element carbon. His plan also accounts for our requirements for inorganic compounds — those not bound to carbon—usually referred to as dietary minerals and trace elements. Inorganic compounds we require in amounts greater than 100 milligrams per day are called minerals; those we need in amounts less than 100 milligrams per day are called trace elements.

Secrets Of An Optimal Nutrition Program!

PROTEINS, the building blocks of life, should come from a variety of sources to insure the availability of all the key amino acids. About 125 grams of protein should be eaten per day, about twice the RDA level.

MINERALS, inorganic compounds essential to good health, are often overlooked. For example, a survey by Dr. J. Matsovinovic, published in the *Journal of the American Medical Association*, shows that 3% of American males and 11% of American females display obvious signs of clinical hyperthyroidism as a result of a deficiency of iodine, even though this type of deficiency was thought to be virtually wiped out in the early days of this century. An iodine intake of at least 50 micrograms per day is essential to maintain the body's production of thyroxine, an enzyme that controls metabolism. In contrast with the Matsovinovic study, Cheraskin's healthy dentists and their families consumed an average of 0.5 milligram of iodine daily—FIVE TIMES THE RDA LEVEL!

Most minerals we consume are stored in our body tissues, so it's important to guard against becoming too enthusiastic and raising intake to dangerous levels. Even so, Cheraskin found an increasing intake of essential minerals—such as calcium, copper, iron, magnesium, manganese, selenium and zinc—paralleled an increase in overall health and a decrease in reported symptoms.

VITAMINS, as we have seen, are not completely understood, even by many so-called experts. The government's RDAs are merely estimates of the amounts needed to prevent full-blown deficiency diseases. Much exciting research on vitamins is being conducted today, but much has already been learned.

In just one example, it is estimated that less than 20% of the U.S. population eats enough fresh fruits and vegetables to reach the RDA of 5000 I.U. (international units) of vitamin A. Cheraskin's studies have demonstrated that the maximum health benefit from vitamin A is reached not at the 5000 I.U. RDA level, but at 33,000 I.U.–NEARLY SEVEN TIMES AS MUCH! This is truly a tragedy for our national health, especially when you consider that the National Cancer Institute has shown that beta-carotene—another form of vitamin A—can arrest development of certain forms of cancer.

Dr. Cheraskin's results continue to show that RDA vitamin levels are inadequate to maintain optimum health. His healthy subjects took in 9 milligrams of thiamine (vitamin B_1), or EIGHT TIMES THE RDA—and 115 milligrams of niacin, about SIX TO SEVEN TIMES THE RDA! Since the B vitamins are critical to brain function, what toll is our national deficiency of these essential vitamins taking on our abilities to think clearly and stay free of mental fatigue?

BIOFLAVONOIDS are a less well known group of nutrients that appear essential for optimal health.

Vitamins' Assistants!

Scientists have long recognized that vitamins and minerals acting alone do not always have the effects that the same nutrients appear to have when consumed as part of the diet. For example, vitamin C in its pure state does not cure bleeding gums, but vitamin C consumed as lemon juice has that effect. Clearly, something ELSE must be at work that unlocks the power of vitamin C, and scientists have been trying to track down this link for decades.

In 1980, French scientists made a breakthrough when they discovered a compound that appears to protect cell walls in plants. It is found in the rind of citrus fruits, in the bark of most trees and in woody shrubs.

This class of substances, known as PAC or pycnogenols, are most commonly called bioflavonoids and act like a "vitamin's vitamin" to help unlock the ability of vitamins to increase our health.

Improve Your Attitude
With Proper Nutrition!

Dr. Cheraskin has clearly demonstrated that adequate nutrition can affect mental attitude and disposition as well as physical health. He describes a 50-year-old male patient with a "rotten" disposition. The man told the doctor he was "shy and sensitive" but complained of a "violent temper" and of being "nervous under pressure." His sour disposition was destroying his personal and professional relationships.

A few months after beginning Dr. Cheraskin's optimum nutrition plan, the patient reported his mood swings and temper tantrums were eliminated. And he could perform better under pressure, such as discussing sensitive issues with his boss without becoming nervous.

Diet Alone Can't Insure Optimum Health!

Dr. Cheraskin's research established the vital importance of diet in maintaining optimum health, but it also showed that diet alone can't insure we get all the nutrients we need and get them in the right balance—and that some elements of our diet can be bad for our overall health.

Refined carbohydrates—sugar, for example—were shown to influence health. Those who reported eating the most sugar also reported the most symptoms, while those who reported eating the least sugar also reported the fewest symptoms of ill health.

But perhaps even more important, Dr. Cheraskin found that some people in his survey were getting too much of one nutrient and at the same time not enough of another as a result of their eating habits. Rarely did he discover, even among his sophisticated sampling of highly trained medical professionals and their families, people who chose a diet optimized for their health. And, he realized, even if you eat the proper foods and eat them in the right combinations, you would need more food than you could eat to get the proper nutrition.

One reason is that processing, packaging, freezing, and cooking destroy many of the biologically available nutrients in the foods we eat, compared to the same foods before they are processed. Our lifestyle often doesn't allow us to prepare foods in the manner that preserves their maximum nutritional value. Yet the stresses and pressures of modern life—such as exposure to pollutants and our ever faster pace—actually can INCREASE our requirements for certain nutrients.

Why It's Vital To Supplement!

Dr. Cheraskin concluded that to insure the best health, top energy and performance, better mental functions, and your best possible appearance, you should take supplemental nutrients. Because it is nearly impossible to determine how much nutrition we receive from the food we eat, Dr. Cheraskin advocates taking supplements that provide all of the vitamins, minerals and trace nutrients his research demonstrates we need daily.

Other researchers concur. A team at the University of California reports their study of over 11,000 people demonstrates that supplementing the diet with vitamin C alone can add more than six healthy years to the life expectancy of men and a smaller number of "bonus" years for women.

Dr. Ranjit Chandra of the Memorial University of Newfoundland in St. John's found that senior citizens receiving vitamin and mineral supplements reported 40% to 50% fewer days of illness than seniors who received placebos.

Some of the vitamins on Cheraskin's optimum list are anti-oxidants that combat free radicals that can accelerate aging. Many scientists around the world believe these nutrients are not enough by themselves to counteract the effect of free radicals. In addition to the nutrients on this optimum list, you should also take more powerful anti-oxidants including SOD, GH3, ACF and glutathione.

Here, then, are the daily vitamin and mineral supplements that Dr. Cheraskin's work suggests you need to maintain your peak health.

OPTIMUM DAILY VITAMIN AND MINERAL SUPPLEMENTATION

VITAMINS

Vitamin A (retinol palmitate)	5000 I.U.
Vitamin A (beta-carotene)	15,000 I.U.
Vitamin C	2000 I.U.
Vitamin E (d-alpha tocopherol)	400 I.U.
Vitamin D (cholecalciferol)	1000 I.U.
Pantothenic acid	70 mg
Vitamin B_1 (thiamine)	50 mg
Vitamin B_2 (riboflavin)	10 mg
Vitamin B_3 (niacinamide)	45 mg
Vitamin B_6 (pyridoxine HCL)	50 mg
Vitamin B_{12} (cyanocobalamin)	50 mcg
Folic acid	400 mcg
Biotin	300 mcg
Choline	250 mg
Inositol	30 mg

MINERALS

Calcium (carbonate, hydrolyzed protein chelate)	1000 mg
Magnesium (oxide-chelate and gluconate)	500 mg
Potassium (amino acid complex)	50 mg
Iron (chelate)	18 mg
Zinc (picolinate)	30 mg
Manganese (chelate)	10 mg
Copper (chelate)	3 mg
Iodine (kelp)	75 mcg
Silicon (chelate)	20 mg
Selenium (chelate)	100 mcg
Chromium (picolinate)	300 mcg
Molybdenum (chelate)	150 mcg

BIOFLAVONOIDS

Lemon bioflavonoids	60 mg
Quercetin (saphora japonica)	30 mg
Rutin (*saphora japonica*)	25 mg
Heseperidin (citrus)	10 mg

Let's take a closer look at these vital nutrients and see just how each is important for your good health.

Vitamin A—The Infection Fighter!

At one time hailed as the "anti-infective vitamin", later cheered as a cancer fighter, today vitamin A's immune system stimulating properties are again grabbing headlines. It is recognized as a curative and restorative for the skin and is the basis of the highly publicized drug Retin-A, used to fight acne, wrinkles and balding.

Long recognized as essential for human health, vitamin A is available in meats, carrots, cantaloupes, sweet potatoes and many other fruits and vegetables, especially those with a yellow orange color.

Vitamin A is needed for night vision, regulation of cell development and reproduction. Deficiencies can cause changes in the skin and mucous membranes, and possibly lead to pre-cancerous conditions.

In laboratory tests with animals, vitamin A supplements have been shown to increase immunity with increased antibody activity, improve acceptance of skin grafts and lead to faster production of a variety of disease fighting cells. Giving vitamin A to children in Third World countries where measles is still common has been shown to cut the death rate from the disease by 35%.

Very high doses of preformed vitamin A—given for a short time—are prescribed by doctors for cancer patients undergoing radiation and chemotherapy treatments. The vitamin A reduces the destructive consequences of these immunosuppressive therapies.

Preformed vitamin A can be toxic in large doses, but the precursor, beta-carotene, does not appear to be toxic even in substantial, sustained dosages of as much as 500,000 I.U. daily. Because of the well-known toxicity of preformed vitamin A supplementation, many doctors warn their patients away from vitamin A, completely ignoring the far safer beta-carotene form.

Beta-carotene used in the same circumstances in animal experiments has much the same beneficial effect with few of the unwanted toxic side effects of preformed vitamin A. Large population studies suggest beta-carotene has protective effects working directly against various forms of cancer, including those of the bladder, larynx, esophagus, stomach, colon/rectum and prostate.

In healthy males with normal immune functions, research has shown that supplemental beta-carotene increases the number of T-lymphocytes, or "helper" cells, in the immune system. And in the laboratory, the addition of beta-carotene stimulated neutrophiles immune cells to more effectively fight off the yeast infection *Candida albicans*, commonly known as thrush, which attacks AIDS patients and others with weakened immune systems.

Vitamin C—An Anti-Cancer Miracle?

So many claims have been made for vitamin C (also known as ascorbic acid) that it's sometimes hard to know how much to believe. One thing seems certain: there are more people taking vitamin C supplements today than any other nutrient—with some surveys showing that as much as HALF the U.S. population takes vitamin C daily. No doubt much of the popularity of vitamin C can be attributed to the efforts and visibility of its most famous champion, the Nobel Prize winner Dr. Linus Pauling. For decades, Dr. Pauling has touted the abilities of vitamin C to prevent and alleviate colds and to prevent cancer.

Like the "limeys" of the old British Navy, we can get vitamin C from many fresh fruits and vegetables. Citrus fruits in particular are recognized as a rich source of vitamin C. No studies, however, have demonstrated that

have been relieved by vitamin E (taken under a doctor's supervision) include muscle weakness, abnormal eye movements, loss of reflexes, restriction of field of vision, unsteady gait and loss of muscle mass. Certain forms of diarrhea can also be symptomatic of a vitamin E deficiency.

Recently, several studies have revealed that children with epilepsy have low vitamin E levels. Supplements of vitamin E help to control seizures among these patients.

One side effect of the long-term use of major tranquilizers used to reduce psychotic behavior is the neurological condition known as tardive dyskinesia, which is characterized by involuntary movements. A double blind study demonstrated that vitamin E reduced the frequency by as much as 43%.

Research concentrating on the immune system demonstrated a correlation between the level of vitamin E and optimum immunity in mice. And a human study linked low blood levels of vitamin E to an increased risk of lung cancer.

Vitamin E Has Many Functions!

There are a number of theories on just how vitamin E works to stimulate the immune system. One school of thought continues to investigate the nutrient's antioxidant properties, while an alternative approach suggests vitamin E can block prostaglandins, chemicals that reduce immune responses. Still another beneficial action of vitamin E is its ability to protect cell membranes, reducing their susceptibility to attack by viruses and other pathogens.

Long term vitamin E therapy has also been shown to be effective against narrowing of the arteries, such as the painful condition of the calves called termittent claudication. In one study, relief from persistent cramping of the legs and feet was reported by 82% of 125 patients given less than 300 I.U. of vitamin E daily. Five hundred I.U. of vitamin E per day has also been shown to elevate blood levels of HDL cholesterol—the so-called good cholesterol—by 14%. Other studies have indicated vitamin

E supplementation can be helpful against conditions ranging from precancerous breast lesions to life-threatening blood clots.

Vitamin E protects us from ozone and nitrogen dioxide, both components of smog, cancer causing nitrosamines, radiation and chemotherapies and even the toxins in cigarette smoke.

There is also experimental evidence that vitamin E can increase the ability of the mineral selenium to inhibit breast cancer and to ward off the formation of other types of tumors. Low blood levels of vitamin E have been linked to a greater risk of lung cancer.

Some doctors use vitamin E, separately or in combination with other therapies, to treat fibrocystic diseases of the breast, such as mammary dysplasia, a precancerous condition. Some 70% of women treated with 600 milligrams of vitamin E daily reported relief. And Vitamin E is also used to treat the symptoms of PMS (premenstrual syndrome), with 400 I.U. being effective in one double blind study.

Vitamin D—Can The Sunshine Vitamin Cure Cancer?

Unique among vitamins, vitamin D is the only nutrient whose active form is actually a hormone produced in the skin from the ultraviolet rays of the sun. Vitamin D can also be taken as a supplement.

Vitamin D is available in trace amounts in some foods, principally fatty fish, liver, egg yolks and milk fat. Because these foods are often avoided by people seeking optimum health, and because it is minimal even in these dietary sources, vitamin D is commonly supplemented.

In the years before most milk commercially available in the United States was fortified with vitamin D_2 (one of the nutrient's two major forms), children with vitamin D deficiencies often were afflicted with rickets, a disease characterized by defective mineralization of growing bones. Luckily, this disease is now quite uncommon, but it does demonstrate the importance of vitamin D in the regulation of calcium metabolism and its promotion of calcium absorption from the gut.

But just because rickets seems a thing of the past doesn't mean that we can forget about vitamin D, because exciting new studies have shown it to have remarkable powers to optimize our health. For example, much work is being conducted on the role of vitamin D in the proliferation and differentiation of cells. This research is already having an impact on the understanding and treatment of cancer. It also appears vitamin D is crucial to the process of immunomodulation, with effects in the prevention and treatment of infectious diseases. And vitamin D's influence on the fluidity of cell membranes is related to nearly all biological processes, including aging.

Some of the latest research suggests vitamin D protects against colorectal and breast cancer and is beneficial in the treatment of other forms of cancer. Some researchers even speculate that chronic vitamin D deficiency can ultimately lead to breast or colon cancer late in life.

Elderly Need More Vitamins!

The elderly are at special risk for a deficiency of vitamin D. They may have too little exposure to sunlight, consume inadequate amounts of foods containing vitamin D, or take drugs that interfere with metabolism of the vitamin. Alcoholics, people with malabsorption problems, and those who live in regions with little sunlight can also be vulnerable to vitamin D deficiency.

Since 1985, the evidence has been mounting that vitamin D protects against cancer. Scientists who compared a map of the United States with rates of death from colon and breast cancer discovered that these deaths are most common in areas with the least sunshine.

Also in 1985, a team at the University of California, San Diego, published startling findings based on the 19 year long Western Electric Health Study. This study, begun in 1957, followed 2000 men who worked at Western Electric's Hawthorne Works in Chicago. The data revealed the only major way men who later develop colorectal cancer differed from those who didn't, was that those who came down with cancer consumed much lower amounts of foods containing vitamin D and calcium.

Confirming these findings, scientists have found that vitamin D inhibits the growth of human colon cancer cells, breast cancer cells, leukemia cells, malignant melanoma cells, and lymphoma cells in test tubes. It also prevents known carcinogens from causing tumors on mouse skin and inhibits the growth of a common form of eye cancer both when it is applied to tumors and WHEN INCLUDED IN THE DIET.

As if all this weren't enough, vitamin D has also been shown to be effective in treating the skin disorder psoriasis. A Boston University scientist tried vitamin D on the reddish, scaly patches caused by the abnormal growth of skin cells characteristic of this condition. All the patients in the study had normal levels of vitamin D, but when its active form was used as a supplement, many reported sympton relief. Sunlight is also known to help the condition.

Long before the age of wonder drugs, victims of tuberculosis went to the mountains for a rest cure. There, the fresh air and sunshine helped many. Today, we understand that some of these patients were probably suffering from a deficiency of vitamin D and that the sunlight was instrumental in their cure. Two groups of researchers, working independently, have found that the active form of vitamin D stimulates human macrophages—a type of white blood cell—to attack the bacterium that causes tuberculosis and to slow down and even stop its growth.

Pantothenic Acid—A New Fountain of Youth!

Parts of the B vitamin complex, pantothenic acid and its cousin pantetheine are vital to human metabolism. We depend on them for the proper production of adrenal hormones and for the production of energy. All manner of claims have been made for these nutrients, from protection against cardiovascular disease and elevated cholesterol, to reduction of the negative effects of aging.

Organ meats and whole grain cereals are known to be dietary sources of pantothenic acid.

There is inconclusive scientific evidence to support the claim that pantothenic acid heightens energy and athletic ability, but many people enthusiastically claim it does. A number of studies do point to the benefits of pantothenic acid supplementation to arthritis patients. Interestingly, in one study rheumatoid arthritis sufferers were found to have below normal levels of pantothenic acid in their blood. When they received supplements, they reported a marked reduction in the discomfort caused by their arthritic conditions, but the symptoms soon returned when supplements were stopped. In 1980, the *General Practitioner Researcher* ran a study that revealed "highly significant effects" of oral pantothenic acid in reducing stiffness, pain and overall disability among rheumatoid arthritis patients.

The vitamin also seems to stimulate cell growth in the healing process. In studies with animals, surgical wounds healed faster in those treated with pantothenic acid supplements.

And recent experimental evidence suggests that pantotheine can help detoxify alcohol in the bloodstream. It appears to have an effect against the component acetaldehyde, a major factor in the ravages of long-term alcohol abuse.

In experiments with rats, pantothenic acid deficiencies have led to graying hair and hair loss. This has encouraged a claim that the vitamin can cure hair loss in humans and reverse the graying of hair. While there is some evidence that pantothenic acid may be effective in these uses, there is no current scientific evidence to prove it.

Similarly, laboratory studies with mice suggest that pantothenic acid may help re-energize old cells and extend their life span, as well as diminish the "age spots" that can appear on the skin. In this experiment, mice given supplements of pantothenic acid lived 20% longer than mice who didn't receive the supplement.

Vitamin B₁—The Drinking Man's Vitamin!

Serious vitamin deficiencies are not a widespread problem in most developed countries—with the exception of vitamin B₁. More adults are deficient in this vitamin than in any other. The reason: the high rate of alcoholism. Alcohol is especially destructive to thiamine—vitamin B¹—in the body.

Among alcoholics, vitamin B₁ deficiency is common. Not only does the alcohol prevent the vitamin stored in the tissue from being converted to its active form, but alcoholics often also eat a diet low in vitamin B₁ to begin with. Large supplemental doses can usually help alcoholics with B₁ deficiencies.

All foods contain some vitamin B₁. Whole grains, brown rice, seafood and beef are rich sources. Highly refined and milled foods, such as polished white rice, are robbed of their vitamin B₁.

In the body, vitamin B₁ is an integral part of the process of converting blood sugar into energy. It is involved in essential metabolic reactions in nervous tissue, the heart, new cell formation and is vital in the maintenance of both smooth and skeletal muscles. If a vitamin B₁ deficiency persists, the deficiency disease beriberi is likely to be the result, with its classic symptoms of confusion, visual disturbances, partial paralysis, and trouble walking. Another form of the disease affects the heart and circulatory system and can lead to death.

A Heart Victim!

Other symptoms of a deficiency of vitamin B₁ are uneven heartbeat, shortness of breath, low blood pressure, chest and abdominal pain, kidney failure, and ultimately heart failure and death. Except for the last, all these symptoms can be effectively treated and reversed with vitamin B₁ supplements.

In experiments using dogs, vitamin B₁ has been beneficial in treating heart attacks, with injections stimulating contractions and decreasing the heart's demand for oxygen. Russian researchers have reported similar results with humans.

One type of anemia responds to large doses of vitamin B_1. Although most people with this condition have what appears to be normal levels of the vitamin, their conditions improve when treated with relatively high doses of up to 100 milligrams per day.

Lead is one of the most common—and most damaging—pollutants in our environment. Vitamin B_1 has been shown to be effective against the high toxicity of lead and levels of the poison in the tissues of experimental animals.

Vitamin B_2—The Athletic Vitamin!

Vitamin B_2, also known as riboflavin, acts together with an enzyme to help produce energy and also to protect against free radical damage. It is a powerful antioxidant. Water soluble, vitamin B_2 cannot be stored in the body and must be replaced continuously to avert a deficiency. Active people, athletes, and, particularly, women often need extra vitamin B_2.

Some of the best dietary sources of vitamin B_2 are milk, cheese, and yogurt. Deficiencies are found in people who eat an unbalanced diet, especially the elderly and alcoholics. vitamin B_2 can also be destroyed by certain drugs, including tranquilizers.

Cracks around the mouth and lips, a reddening of the tongue, and eczema of the face and genitals can all be symptomatic of a deficiency of vitamin B_2. Riboflavin is thought to be important in the absorption of iron, so many people deficient in B_2 are also anemic.

Deficiencies of riboflavin have been linked with cancer of the esophagus. The growth of precancerous cells in the esophagus has been reduced with B_2 supplements.

Vitamin B₃—The Cholesterol Buster!

Vitamin B₃ is a hot topic in medical circles these days because one of its forms is rapidly being accepted as a preferred treatment for lowering blood cholesterol levels. Safer and apparently more effective than multi-million dollar anticholesterol drugs, vitamin B₃ has fewer side effects and COSTS 40 TIMES LESS THAN THE DESIGNER DRUG!

This miracle nutrient is acknowledged to significantly reduce the risk of death among people who have had heart attacks. And many claim it can treat and even cure schizophrenia. What's more, it is recognized as a detoxifying agent able to rid the body of many poisons, including narcotics.

A true vitamin powerhouse, B₃ is available in lean meats and poultry. Various forms of supplements are also commonly available. As niacin, vitamin B₃ can cause a flushing of the face and neck, itching, and dizziness. In the form of niacinamide, these unpleasant side effects will be avoided.

Cuts Heart Attacks By 30%!

As little as two grams a day are now known to reduce blood levels of cholesterol and triglycerides, which can form deposits inside blood vessels and lead to heart attacks and strokes. The Coronary Project Research Group's major 1975 study found that B₃ not only reduces cholesterol, but cuts back the likelihood of subsequent heart attacks by almost 30%.

As if this weren't amazing enough, follow-up work to the famous Coronary Drug Project study showed that heart attack patients who took vitamin B₃ instead of a placebo lived longer and had fewer later medical problems in every category: second heart attacks, other cardiovascular diseases, cancer, and "all others." The patients who got the vitamin treatment were also less likely to die than those treated with major anti-cholesterol pharmaceuticals. In fact, the expensive drugs were demonstrated to be no more effective than the placebo in preventing death—in other words, they were as good as nothing (but a lot more expensive)!

Vitamin B_3 in moderate doses has also been shown to increase blood levels of HDL (the so-called "good cholesterol") by 33%.

Many have claimed remarkable success using vitamin B_3 to remove toxins from the system, often in a regimen that includes sauna baths and running. The Foundation for Advancement in Science and Education, based in Los Angeles, confirmed the results of this process as practiced by the drug rehabilitation program Narconon, as well as a simultaneous reduction in cholesterol levels.

There have been claims that vitamin B_3 reduces addicts' craving for alcohol and drugs, but they have not been proven. Similarly, vitamin B_3 has also been reported to reduce high blood pressure.

The assertions that mental illness such as schizophrenia can be cured with vitamin B_3 probably originated with its use to treat the deficiency disease pellagra, caused by a lack of B vitamins and typified by symptoms including dementia. No adequate proof of niacin's effectiveness against mental illnesses not caused by a B vitamin deficiency has been reported, but some mental health professionals claim success with this treatment.

Vitamin B_6—The Super Immunity Builder!

Without vitamin B_6, more than 60 essential enzymes could not function properly. Normal nucleic acid and protein synthesis would grind to a halt. And the multiplication of cells—especially red blood cells and cells of the immune system—would become impossible. The nervous system and brain would cease to function properly as production of neurotransmitters broke down. Deficiency of vitamin B_6 leads to anemia, nervous disorders and skin problems. Women are in particular need of B_6 if they're on the Pill, if they're pregnant; and when they're dealing with the effects of premenstrual syndrome. There's even new reason to believe B_6 has cancer fighting powers.

But most important of all is the function of vitamin B_6 in maintaining our immunity. Of all the B vitamins, B_6 may be most crucial for maintaining a vigorous immune system. B_6 is found in meats, whole grains and brewer's yeast.

Elderly people, alcoholics, lab animals, and human volunteers have all demonstrated that a lack of adequate vitamin B_6 leads to a severe compromise of the immune system. Both AIDS victims and cancer patients show low levels of B_6.

Supplements of B_6 have boosted immunity among elderly patients and reduced cancerous tumor growth. Vitamin B_6 applied in a cream to melanomas—skin cancers that are highly resistant to treatment— caused reduction and even disappearance of cancerous nodules.

In one study, women treated with vitamin B_6 for the symptoms of premenstrual tensions (headaches, weight gain, irritability) not only enjoyed relief from their symptoms, but many with fertility problems also were able to conceive. In another study of B_6's effect on premenstrual syndrome, women reported it reduced nausea, depression and anxiety.

For decades it's been well-established that a deficiency of B_6 can lead to convulsions and problems with peripheral nerves. And it's been used for forty years to treat convulsions in newborns with metabolic disorders.

Alleviate Carpal Tunnel Syndrome!

More recently, vitamin B_6 has been used successfully to treat carpal tunnel syndrome, a painful compression of the nerves in the wrist that can cause pain and a pins-and-needles sensation extending into the hand as well. While most other treatments are ineffective, 100 to 200 milligrams of B_6 daily usually clears up the condition within about three months.

Diabetics with abnormal metabolism of the amino acid triptophan and the related intolerance of glucose, one of the basic sugars, have been helped with B_6. For some diabetics, B_6 supplements can even reduce the need for insulin.

Many women who use oral contraceptives experience the same type of abnormal triptophan metabolism as diabetics. About 5 milligrams of vitamin B_6 can usually reverse this situation and return glucose tolerance to normal.

Vitamin B12—The Super Energy Secret

Because so many claims have been made about B12 over the years, many in the medical establishment have pooh-poohed it as a modern day snake oil. They grudgingly agree that it is essential in humans for healthy nerve tissues. And they acknowledge deficiency of B12 can cause problems ranging from nerve disorders and brain damage to anemia. But only in recent years have its more remarkable properties been gaining credence within the medical establishment.

In the diet, vitamin B12 is available in fish, dairy products, organ meats such as liver and kidney, eggs, beef, and pork.

Until fairly recently, it was difficult to accurately diagnose a vitamin B12 deficiency. If one of the most common symptoms—anemia—was not present, doctors did not believe there could be an inadequate supply of B12. But with today's more sensitive tests, it is possible to discover that people are suffering from too little vitamin B12 even if they are not anemic.

As a treatment for stress, fatigue and recovery from trauma, vitamin B12 certainly benefits people with pernicious anemia, but more medical doctors today are admitting that injections of B12 appear to have equally dramatic positive effects on patients who do not show signs of B12 deficiency. One doctor wrote in *Medical World* that, like "...thousands of other physicians..." he was convinced B12 can help speed recovery from viral and bacterial infections as well as surgery. Like others, he reports it helps restore appetite and a higher energy level.

B12 is used to treat various neuropsychiatric problems and to prevent mental deterioration, especially in the elderly who are likely to have B12 deficiencies. Of 39 patients treated with vitamin B12 for neurologic problems such as abnormal gait, memory loss, poor reflexes, weakness, fatigue and psychiatric disorders, all showed improvement—and some showed dramatic improvement. It is effective in treating neurologic damage.

Vitamin B_{12} has also been demonstrated to help counteract the consequences of cigarette smoking. It has long been recognized that components in cigarette smoke reduce the levels of B_{12} and folic acid in the cells of the lungs and bronchioles. In one experiment, 73 longtime heavy smokers were studied. They all had developed precancerous tissue, but none had cancer. They were split into two groups, one being given B_{12} and folic acid, and the other a placebo. Four months later, the treated smokers had significantly fewer precancerous cells than the control group.

Recently, a new study demonstrated that B_{12} blocks allergic reactions to the sulfites used as additives in some foods and wines. These reactions include headache, congestion, running nose and bronchial spasms.

Sulfite sensitive subjects were given 2000 micrograms of B_{12}, then exposed to sulfites. All except one avoided any allergic reaction. This test, repeated successfully with a control group, suggests B_{12} can help others who suffer from allergies.

Folic Acid—Can the DNA Builder Help Smokers?

A key player in some of the most basic metabolic processes in our bodies, folic acid is essential in the synthesis of DNA (the blueprint for cell growth and reproduction). It has also recently been promoted as being able to prevent certain cancers and birth defects.

Folic acid is available in fresh leafy green vegetables, yeasts and liver, among other dietary sources.

A deficiency of folic acid can show up as a type of anemia termed megaloblastic anemia whose symptoms include a feeling of overall weakness, tiring easily, irritability and cramps. Deficiencies can be caused by poor diet (common among the elderly) and malabsorption problems. Pregnant women are at risk of folic acid deficiency, as are those who are deficient in vitamin B_{12}. Some drugs and blood conditions can also cause folic acid deficiencies.

Studies dating back to the 1970s demonstrated that precancerous cervical cells could be eliminated with large doses of folic acid. National Cancer Institute researchers in 1986 found that smokers showing abnormal bronchial cells known to be prone to becoming cancerous had depressed levels of folic acid in their blood. Scientists at the University of Alabama, reported in 1988, were able to reduce this type of precancerous growth in smokers with a combination of folic acid and vitamin B_{12}.

Too little folic acid increases smokers' susceptibility to cancerous changes in the lung tissue. It can also increase the malignancy potential of cancers in other parts of the body. A University of Vermont researcher reported not long ago that mouse melanoma (skin cancer) cells low in folic acid were much more likely to spread when injected into mice than similar cells with normal folic acid levels. The same study demonstrated that the cancer cells low in folic acid were more likely to spread than those with normal amounts of folic acid even after their folic acid deficiency was brought up to normal levels. This suggests that something irreversible happens to the cells during the time they were deficient in folic acid. Knowing the part folic acid plays in DNA formation, it is suspected this lethal change is breakage of the chromosomes due to folic acid starvation.

Folic Acid Is Important
For Pregnant Women!

More and more is learned about human chromosomes every day. So far, at least 51 sites have been identified along the chromosome where breakage is likely to occur—and twenty of these places, when damaged, are associated with the formation of cancer. Test tube studies have shown cells are far more likely to have breaks in the DNA chain—including at these known cancer-stimulating sites—when they are grown with too little folic acid. Based on what is now understood, some scientists believe that oral supplementation of folic acid may lower the risk of developing cancer.

Folic acid is also used with pregnant women to help prevent neural tube defects that can cause mental retardation in their babies.

Like Down's Syndrome, Fragile X Syndrome is an inherited disorder of males that is an identified cause of mental retardation. French scientists reported in 1981 that oral supplements of folic acid were effective at improving some of the behavior abnormalities characteristic of retarded boys with Fragile X Syndrome.

A 1986 study of a similar group of boys showed that 10 milligrams a day of folic acid resulted in some improvement in their behavior. Prepubertal boys also showed some increase in IQ, but older boys did not. Studies continue with this population, but evidence so far shows the benefits are most like to been seen among younger children.

Dr. Kurt Oster and others use folic acid to treat arteriosclerosis. His treatment for patients with arteriosclerotic heart disease is folic acid at two times the RDA, which he reports prevents recurrent heart attacks and also reduces angina (pain in the heart) and the need for the common anti-angina drug, nitroglycerine.

Limited tests have also shown folic acid to be beneficial among the elderly in alleviating the symptoms of peripheral nerve diseases. Intravenous folic acid leads to improved vision in less than an hour, but the effects are short-lived. Elderly diabetic patients given folic acid orally also noticed improved vision and skin temperature. These tests suggest that folic acid may help by opening up blood vessels and allowing increased collateral circulation.

Biotin—The Hair Salon Molecule!

A water-soluble B vitamin, biotin is just now beginning to be studied. Nuts, whole grains, milk, vegetables, organ meats, and brewer's yeast are all good dietary sources of biotin. Biotin deficiency is rare, but when it is seen its primary symptoms are baldness, dry flaky skin and rashes in the nose or mouth.

Raw egg white contains a substance that acts as an antivitamin and appears to destroy biotin. People who consume a lot of raw eggs are at risk of having this substance bind to biotin and thus prevent its absorption by the body. People on long term oral antibiotic therapy are also at risk for biotin deficiency.

Luckily, the baldness that can come from biotin deficiency—even when caused by strict dieting—can be reversed with supplementation.

Many people believe that biotin can promote healthy hair and help prevent graying and baldness. Numerous hair products contain biotin. It remains to be seen whether these theories can stand up to scientific study, but at least one claim about biotin's effects on the hair has been shown to be true.

Children with unruly, "uncombable" hair that insists on sticking out in all directions in a profusion of cowlicks have been helped with biotin. The mechanism by which biotin tames the uncontrollable hair is not understood—but it works.

Because biotin is required for the metabolism of the branched chain amino acids valine, isoleucine and leucine, which some believe can enhance athletic performance, biotin supplementation has been recommended those wishing to improve their strength and stamina.

Choline!

For years one of the most popular—and controversial—dietary supplements was lecithin. Many claims have been made about this nutrient's ability to fight cardiovascular disease and boost energy. But as scientific knowledge of nutritional chemistry grows, the mystery surrounding lecithin and its molecular brethren which include the nutrient choline, has begun to clear up.

New evidence shows that choline can be important in treating major nerve, psychiatric, and infectious diseases—and may yet be beneficial for victims of cardiovascular disease.

Choline (from the chemical compound, phosphatidylcholine) is readily available in the diet, because it's found in all plant and meats. Egg yolks, soybeans, cauliflower and cabbage are good sources. It also is one of the very few substances used as a food additive that actually has nutritional value.

The most recent findings suggest that choline elevates the HDL cholesterol (good cholesterol) level. In addition, injections of choline lower blood pressure while choline taken orally doesn't.

Choline also seems to affect memory loss and other diseases of the nervous system. In 1980, *Science Magazine* reported that choline improved memory in mice. While choline-rich diets also improved memory in animal experiments, but choline-deficient diets appeared to lead to memory loss. People who take drugs that destroy choline (including antihistamines and some anti-depressants) develop short-term memory loss. Some experiments on humans indicate that choline can improve short-term memory. Early tests suggest it may help the memory—and mood— of some Alzheimer's patients as well.

Diseases that result in abnormal muscular movements and that are caused by abnormalities of the neurotransmitter system, including Parkinson's disease and Huntington's disease, can be treated effectively with choline.

Mood disorders, such as manic depression, have also been treated with choline. This therapy is much safer—as well as much cheaper—than lithium, which is a standard treatment for depression and other manic symptoms (and which often doesn't work).

There have been a number of recent reports in medical literature, including an article in the *Journal of Czech Medicine*, suggesting that choline can be effective against viral hepatitis Type A and Type B. It helped provide a quicker end to symptoms and a shorter time for a return to normal liver cell functioning together with fewer relapses. It is believed that choline works by repairing the membranes of liver cells.

Research at King's College Hospital and Medical School in Great Britain confirms the effectiveness of choline containing substances against active hepatitis of the type caused by the virus once known as non-A non-B (also known as hepatitis C). Similar results were reported in studies in Italy and Nigeria.

Another choline containing substance—AL 721—has been proven to inhibit the replication of the AIDS virus in the laboratory. It is being used clinically in an experimental treatment for AIDS. AL 721 has been shown to lessen withdrawal symptoms of morphine addicted mice in laboratory studies conducted in Israel in 1982 and may be helpful for human drug addicts.

Inositol—A Nutritional Nerve Tonic!

Another of the little understood nutrients that is a complex form of fatty acid, inositol (or its nutritionally active form, myo-inositol), is known to be linked to messenger molecules within the nervous system, and plays a key role in controlling various cells within the system.

Fruits, nuts, beans, grains and vegetables are good sources of inositol. Fresh fruits and vegetables usually have more available than those that have been processed or frozen.

Many people report that inositol is a natural tranquilizer that relieves anxiety and promotes sleep. It is known that the level of inositol can influence the levels of certain key compounds within brain cells. In any event, inositol is much safer than chemical tranquilizers or sleeping pills.

Diabetics suffer from the disintegration of peripheral nerves as a result of chronic high blood sugar. An investigation of the effects of inositol on this condition showed improved nerve functioning after inositol was taken, compared to those who took a placebo.

Calcium—What's Good For the Goose...

It's been ten years since a National Institute of Health medical panel dropped a bombshell on the American public: Most American women, it reported, aren't getting enough calcium in their diets. Just one consequence of this deficiency is the degenerative disease osteoporosis, which primarily affects elderly women. In all, there are more than 20 million Americans suffering from osteoporosis today.

But the link between calcium and osteoporosis has turned out to be just the tip of the iceberg. Research next suggested calcium is beneficial in preventing cancer and high blood pressure and in lowering cholesterol. And, perhaps most startling of all, scientists estimate that most Americans are getting as little as a third of the calcium they need to maintain optimum health.

Children have long been admonished to drink their milk, and it's good advice, because dairy products, including milk, cheese, ice cream, yogurt and buttermilk, are excellent dietary sources of calcium. It's also plentiful in salmon, green leafy vegetables and tofu.

Most of us remember learning back in grade school that calcium is a major part of our bones and teeth. It is also vital for nerve conduction, heartbeat and other types of muscle contractions, coagulation (clotting) of the blood, the production of biological energy and maintenance of our immune systems. Besides the well-recognized problems of osteoporosis and cavities, severe calcium deficiency can cause abnormal heartbeat, convulsions and dementia.

Antacids containing aluminum, alcohol, cortisone and some special diets (such as those high protein or fiber), can all lead to a calcium deficiency.

The calcium ion is the most sensitive chemical regulator of human cellular activity known. Even the slightest difference in the concentration of calcium can influence our cells and our organs, causing a skipped heartbeat, for example. And if the concentration becomes too high within a cell, toxic oxygen forms will be created and destroy the cell. Magnesium and calcium work together to maintain the proper delicate balance, which suggests that for optimum nutrition, we must have both calcium and magnesium in the proper ratio.

Calcium Very Important As We Get Older!

As we grow older, we can have increasing difficulty absorbing calcium. Sometimes, the elderly don't eat a well-balanced diet or supplement their nutrition intake. In the case of calcium, this is playing with fire! Because the body requires calcium so absolutely for the regulation of its biochemical processes, if there is insufficient calcium in the diet, the body will look for calcium anywhere it can be found—and too often this means that we literally begin digesting our own bones and teeth for the calcium our cells crave! This is the genesis of osteoporosis, as well as other degenerative diseases.

Alas, once bone has been lost this way, it cannot be replaced, so the secret to avoiding osteoporosis is prevention—which means including enough calcium in the diet, before the damage has a chance to occur. The National Institute of Health recommend premenopausal women get one gram of calcium a day before reaching menopause, and 1500 milligrams a day after that.

Colorectal Cancer!

In a 19 year study of men in Chicago, the incidence of colorectal cancer was linked to the amount of vitamin D and calcium in the diet. These findings have been corroborated by statistical studies in four Scandinavian countries.

Following up on this work, men from families known to be prone to developing colorectal cancers were given 1250 milligrams of calcium daily. Within two or three months, the abnormal rates of cell division in their colons had slowed to normal. Other experiments suggest this result may be due to calcium's ability to detoxify carcinogenic bile acids.

A recent double blind study of calcium's effect on high blood pressure confirmed the findings of doctors who noticed that individuals with hypertension have lower levels of calcium in their bodies than do people with normal blood pressure. The experiment showed calcium to be effective at lowering blood pressure, but the extent of the effect varies according to the individual. A daily supplement of 1500 milligrams of calcium produced a significant lowering of blood pressure in most of those tested.

Calcium can protect against cardiovascular disease in two ways. By lowering blood pressure, it lessens the likelihood of heart attacks and strokes. There has been mounting evidence over the last several decades that calcium also acts directly to lower serum cholesterol levels.

Magnesium—The Heart Mineral!

Magnesium is a major component of our bodies. It is concentrated in our bones and in the liquid filling our cells with life itself. It is indispensable to every major biological such as glucose metabolism, the production of cellular energy, synthesizing nucleic acids and proteins.

Magnesium takes part in maintaining the electrical stability of our cells, membrane integrity, muscle contraction, nerve conduction, and the health of our veins. It is part of a delicate balance with calcium in synthesizing the stuff of life and producing energy.

Magnesium is found in meats, seafoods, green vegetables, and dairy products.

A deficiency of magnesium causes loss of appetite, nausea, vomiting, diarrhea, confusion, tremors, loss of coordination and convulsions. Marginal magnesium deficiency is thought to be fairly common. The elderly, those on weight loss diets, diabetics, pregnant women, people who exercise hard, and people who take certain drugs are all at risk.

Medicine now recognizes that even a slight lack of magnesium can cause life-threatening interruptions in the heart's rhythm. And it is thought by some that magnesium supplements can help protect the heart against the starvation caused by clogged arteries.

Studies have correlated the death rate from heart disease caused by blocked arteries with areas of hard and soft water. They've discovered that areas with high concentrations of minerals—including magnesium—in the water are also areas where the death rate from this type of heart disease are low. Evidence has also been presented that the typical American diet is insufficient in magnesium, which may contribute to our very high rate of cardiovascular disease.

Further studies have shown that in some people the cellular level of magnesium can be inadequate, even when blood magnesium levels are normal. This situation can also contribute to cardiovascular diseases, including high blood pressure.

People who have a recurring problem of calcium-oxalate kidney stones have been helped with supplements of magnesium.

For many years, pregnant women experiencing the life-threatening conditions known as pre-eclampsia and eclampsia have been successfully treated with magnesium. Pre-eclampsia's symptoms include protein in the urine, high blood pressure and swelling of the body. It can lead to the much more serious eclampsia, which can involve convulsions, coma, and ultimately death. No one knows precisely how magnesium helps women experiencing this condition, but it is now a standard therapy.

Potassium—Nature's Treatment For High Blood Pressure!

Potassium is one of the most studied nutrients, partly because of its well-known influence on blood pressure. It is also vital in muscle contraction, nerve conduction, the beating of the heart, the production of biological energy, and the synthesis of nucleic acids and proteins, which are the building blocks of life.

Potassium is widely available in an average diet. Some of the best sources are fresh vegetables and fruits. Bananas in particular are known to be a rich source of potassium. Cantaloupes, oranges, avocadoes, raw spinach, raw celery and raw cabbage are also good sources.

A deficiency of potassium shows up as symptoms throughout the body: Fatigue, weakness, and muscle pains are often noted. Even death can occur if a lack of potassium goes uncorrected.

Much has been written about the harmful effects on our bodies of too much salt. Potassium helps to counteract the effects of salt, and it is also helpful in reducing the effects of hypertension that too much salt can produce. Some have suggested that high blood pressure is not caused (or worsened) by too much salt, but by a lack of sufficient potassium.

This idea is supported by a number of studies. In one, researchers assessed vegetarians and non-vegetarians in Tel Aviv, Israel in 1983. Vegetarians are known to have a higher intake of potassium in their diets than meat eaters. Not only was the average blood pressure level lower in the vegetarian group, but among the vegetarians, only 2% had what could be considered high blood pressure, while 26% of the meat eaters were hypertensive. Of all the factors measured in this study—family history, coffee drinking, smoking and even sodium intake—the only real difference was the level of potassium consumed by the vegetarians.

One of the best pieces of news about the connection between potassium and blood pressure is that, while potassium does not appear to have any effect on NORMAL blood pressure, it appears to lower the blood pressure of many people suffering from HIGH blood pressure. Evidence shows that there are considerable individual differences in the way people react to both potassium and salt, and to how they affect blood pressure.

A high level of potassium consumption has also been shown to protect against death from strokes. A 12-year study of older Southern Californians revealed that those with the highest levels of potassium in their diets had fewer deaths from strokes, while those who did experience fatal strokes all consumed lower levels of potassium. It is interesting that the statistics in this study excluded blood pressure, weight, smoking, blood sugar level and other known risk factors for stroke. The ONLY factor that appeared to be different between those who died of strokes and those who avoided strokes was potassium intake.

Vigorous exercise—such as the efforts of an athlete in training—can lead to the loss of potassium through sweat. To counter the consequent symptoms of muscle weakness and fatigue, a supplement of potassium can contribute to improved athletic performance. The best news of all is that a single banana or serving of vegetables is usually enough to make up for the loss and return the athlete's potassium balance to its optimum level.

Iron—The Body's Alchemist!

Alchemists searched for a way to turn base metals in to precious gold. If they had been able to peek inside their own bodies' chemistry, they would have understood that even the simplest "base" metals—such as iron—are more valuable than gold on the cellular level. In fact, without a reliable supply of iron, we would not be able to sustain life at all!

A number of foods provide a good source of iron, but Popeye notwithstanding, spinach is not one of them. Iron is found in meat (especially organ meat such as liver), poultry, fish, and ground soybean hulls.

Iron is essential to the process of burning the food we eat on the cellular level and creating the biological energy that keeps us alive. Iron is also vital to hemoglobin, the part of the blood that carries oxygen to the cells. It's also a part of the process of forming carnitine, which is needed to oxidize fatty acids. And collagen and elastin—two components vital to the integrity of our connective tissue—both require iron in their composition. The immune system likewise needs iron as it fights infections and oxidation damage.

One of the most obvious consequences of a lack of iron is iron deficiency anemia, a condition that was recognized as long ago as the days of the Pharaohs, even though the cause wasn't understood. By the 17th century, Thomas Sydenham was prescribing iron supplements for chlorosis (green sickness), which today we call iron deficiency anemia.

Iron deficiency is fairly common in infants, adolescents and pregnant women. Even without the telltale anemia, iron deficiency can produce symptoms including behavioral problems, fatigue, muscle weakness and an increased susceptibility to infection. Iron deficiency anemia is the most common deficiency disease in the world, affecting at least a billion people.

Iron occurs in two forms: ferrous and ferric. Free (ferrous) iron generates destructive oxygen radicals and is very toxic. Its harmful effects are rare, though, because most dietary iron is tightly bound in biological structures.

An interesting (though fairly unusual) consequence of iron deficiency is a condition called Plummer-Vinson syndrome, in which a membrane grows across the top of the esophagus and prevents swallowing. People with Plummer-Vinson are at increased risk of cancer in the esophagus or stomach. Supplemental iron can eliminate the condition, as well as the cancer risk.

Iron's effect on the immune system is related to its role in the function of the white blood cells. Candida (a yeast infection) and herpes are more likely to strike people who have iron deficiencies. A key enzyme essential to the synthesis of DNA requires iron.

Oxygen free radicals are generally something the body tries to avoid. But, using iron in the process, some types of white blood cells actually create these toxins and aim them as weapons at invading bacteria. The immune system uses iron in another way—by stimulating an enzyme to create iodine to kill bacteria. This same enzyme is found in human milk and is believed to be one way a nursing mother passes resistance to infection along to her baby.

A slight iron deficiency, and even when there is no obvious anemia, can cause significant muscle weakness. And since the heart is a muscle, a lack of iron can affect its performance and lead to symptoms of heart failure. Active people such as runners, and women more than men, are subject to these debilitating symptoms that result from even small iron deficiencies.

Zinc—The Immunity Tonic!

Zinc is widely recognized as a protector of the immune system and a disease fighter in its own right. It has recently also been found to combat a common eye disorder called macular degeneration, which leads to blindness in the elderly. There is increasing evidence that we all may develop a deficiency of zinc as we grow older.

Many foods contain zinc. Some of the best sources are whole grains, brewer's yeast, wheat bran, and wheat germ. Some people believe that seafood and meat supply more easily absorbed forms of zinc than do vegetables.

There are more than 200 human enzymes known to require zinc in order to function. They include the enzymes we need to produce DNA and RNA. Zinc also allows proteins to bind with nucleic acids and is a building block of cell membranes.

Severe zinc deficiencies in developed countries are rare; however, marginally low levels of zinc are thought to be common. Deficiency can lead to growth retardation, poor appetite, malfunctioning sex glands, lethargy, slow healing and abnormalities of sense and perception. Low levels of zinc are also linked to increased susceptibility to infection.

Animals and people with zinc absorption difficulties are prey to a variety of infections, proving zinc's usefulness in protecting the immune system. Low levels of zinc have also been discovered in AIDS patients. Many elderly people whose diets are deficient in zinc, needlessly fall victim to infections. In addition, there is new evidence that a lack of zinc leads to the gradual breakdown of aging immune systems and the increase in various autoimmune disorders of the elderly, such as arthritis.

Because it is known to boost the immune system and is an anti-viral agent, zinc is now being studied as a cold treatment.

Much faster healing of surgical wounds and ulcers has been reported when patients receive zinc supplements. So far, it is unclear if the remarkable increases in the speed of healing and recovery that have been observed are related to a pre-existing deficiency of zinc among the patients tested, or if zinc as a key part of cellular repair is generally effective for all people.

Zinc is closely related to testosterone, the male sex hormone. It has helped to increase male potency and sex drive in men with suboptimal zinc levels.

A topical application of zinc, together with an antibiotic, helps to improve acne even in people who are not obviously deficient in zinc.

Because of their special diets and abnormal metabolisms, diabetics often show symptoms of zinc deficiency. Zinc is also important to the normal functioning of insulin. Many people believe zinc supplements can therefore reduce some of the complications of diabetes.

Until recent times, there has been strong resistance in the medical and pharmaceutical communities to treatments using nutrients. Perhaps the example of zinc in the treatment of a rare condition called Wilson's disease argues the case best. This is an always fatal disease of copper accumulation. Oral zinc has been shown to be effective against the disease with no side effects. The conventional drug therapy, peninillamine, is toxic to many patients, as well as much more expensive than zinc. Here is another instance in which treatment with nutrition is at least as effective, safer and cheaper than treatment with drugs.

Manganese—The Mystery Mineral!

Science knows that manganese makes some of the most basic biological functions possible, including the production of energy. As an antioxidant, manganese may also help to protect us from the toxic effects of some forms of oxygen. But little else is well understood about this enigmatic mineral.

Manganese is available to us in whole grains and nuts, as well as in some fruits and green vegetables, but the amount depends heavily on the level of manganese in the soil where they were grown. Alkaline soils produce vegetable with little manganese content. In grains, manganese tends to concentrate in the bran, which unfortunately is often removed by milling. It is also present in organ meats, shellfish and milk.

Animals are known to develop manganese deficiency, but its role in human nutrition is still shrouded in mystery. Lowering of serum cholesterol levels, impaired blood clotting, dermatitis and changes in hair color occur in humans lacking in manganese, but deficiencies are not commonly seen.

Dietary manganese is low in toxicity, but people exposed to a great deal of it develop a syndrome known as manganese intoxication, or manganese madness. Chilean manganese miners with this condition have the following symptoms: Impulsiveness, heightened sexuality, unaccountable laughter, and hallucinations. These early stage progresses to a state of deep depression and ultimately to symptoms similar to Parkinson's Disease. Like Parkinson's, manganese poisoning is treated with the drug L-dopa.

Manganese has the unusual property of being able to substitute for magnesium in many biochemical processes. When analyzed, tumors typically show decreased levels of manganese, which suggests to some that manganese may play a role—still not understood—in the human degenerative process.

Other possible needs for this mysterious mineral include proper brain function and the synthesis of the neurotransmitter dopamine. Going along with this, there is a school of thought that believes manganese can be useful in the treatment of schizophrenia and some neurological disorders.

Animals deficient in manganese sometimes have reproductive failure. This may be because manganese is involved in the synthesis of sex hormones.

Other animal studies suggest that manganese is needed for the development of normal bone structure, particularly the growth of the matrix of cartilage at the ends of the bones where the formation of new bone tissue takes place. This has suggested manganese as a treatment for osteoarthritis, a theory encouraged by studies showing a significantly lowered level of manganese in women with osteoarthritis.

A large number of unsubstantiated claims have been made for manganese in humans, and investigation continues into our need for this mystery mineral, known to be essential to life itself.

Copper—The Molecular Fire Department!

There is now no question that copper is an essential trace mineral needed for good human health. It is vital to normal respiration. Copper is required (along with iron) for the synthesis of hemoglobin, the substance that carries oxygen in the blood. It is also part of the formation of the protein collagen which holds together bones, tendon, skin and cartilage. Copper is needed in the production of elastin, which makes our blood vessels, lungs and skin flexible. The neurotransmitter norepinephrine, a key messenger in the nervous system, is produced using copper, as is melanin, which gives pigment to our hair and skin and helps protect us from the ultraviolet rays of the sun.

Copper also combines to form enzymes that protect the body from oxidation damage. It is one of the most important blood antioxidants. As if all this isn't enough, copper also prevents polyunsaturated fatty acids in our bodies from turning rancid and contributes to the integrity of cell membranes, so essential to the limitation of the production of free radicals.

Dietary copper is available in animal livers, crustaceans, shellfish, nuts, fruits, oysters, kidney and dried legumes.

The body chemical ceruloplasmin, dependant on copper, is what is known as an acute-phase reactant. The body produces as much as is needed to help combat toxic and infectious agents. Ceruloplasmin acts like the body's fire department—an emergency antioxidant squad rushed to the scene of disaster to quench the cellular fire.

Copper deficiencies are thought to be responsible for lung damage from,emphysema. Other symptoms include anemia, low white blood cell count and loss of bone density. High levels of zinc supplementation can cause copper deficiency over time.

As an anti-cancer agent, copper has been tested in a number of experiments. In one, copper protected rats against chemically induced cancers. In another, chicks were protected against a form of cancer caused by a virus. And in still another, a copper salt protected mice against cancerous tumor formation.

Copper deficiency in young men leads to a significant lowering of the level of HDL in the blood. A supporting experiment in mice shows that a copper/zinc imbalance can increase the risk of heart disease by lowering HDL levels. These and other studies suggest that the ratio of zinc to copper should be balanced at about 10:1.

Copper also appears to have an effect on the immune system. Laboratory rats with copper deficiencies showed a higher mortality rate from salmonella infection than properly nourished rats. Copper deficiencies in mice result in decreased antibody response.

More research into this fascinating nutrient mineral is progressing. As the body's volunteer fire department, we depend on copper for long and healthy lives.

Iodine—The Medicine Cabinet Radiation Protector!

Iodine is rare on land, but plentiful in the sea. It is vital for the production of thyroid hormones, which control the production of energy. Deficiency of iodine results in hypothyroidism—an overall slowing down of the bodily functions.

Iodine is available in seafoods, including sea animals and kelp.

Years ago, iodine deficiency in the United States was rather common, and led to an enlargement of the thyroid (goiter) and the symptoms of chronic fatigue, apathy, dry skin, sensitivity to cold and weight gain.

Luckily, iodine deficiency is relatively rare today because it is now added to table salt.

Unfortunately, we are also now more subject to exposure to unsafe levels of radiation, and here iodine can be protective. Iodine can block the uptake of radioactive iodides by the thyroid. This is effective in preventing the highly toxic effects of radiation on the thyroid, which is particularly vulnerable to attack by radioactive pollutants.

In 1988, a Canadian physician reported that a majority of the women he treated for a painful condition called fibrocystic breasts were completely relieved of their symptoms after being treated with elemental iodine. When the iodine supplement was discontinued, the pain came back, suggesting that this condition is a result of an iodine deficiency.

An iodine containing compound is also used by physicians to help break up mucus in persistently congested breathing tubes when the congestion causes a cough that never quite goes away.

Most familiar is iodine the antiseptic, good for cuts, scrapes and purifying backcountry water.

Silicon—A New Treatment for Arteriosclerosis?

Silicon is one of the most common elements on earth, and is found in the world around us in forms as varied as sand, glass and computer chips. Recently, some have speculated that it may also be a key to reversing arteriosclerosis—hardening of the arteries—in humans.

In the diet, silicon is available in vegetables, whole grains, and seafood.

Studies have revealed that, as we age, the levels of silicon in our arteries and skin decline. French researchers report finding a correlation between the level of silicon in the walls of the human aorta and the development of arteriosclerosis.

Selenium—A Secret Weapon Against Cancer!

In very, very small amounts, selenium can have a major impact on our health. For many years, selenium was ignored as a nutrient because it is highly toxic and because it was thought to be carcinogenic. But recent findings show that not only is it essential for optimum health, but that selenium actually protects against cancer.

Selenium is available in many vegetables including broccoli, cucumbers, onions, garlic and radishes. The selenium content of foods, however, is extremely dependent on the selenium content of the soils where they are grown, and there are considerable regional differences.

Selenium deficiencies are now known to occur in most warm-blooded animals and can cause cataracts, muscular dystrophy, liver disease, infertility, heart problems, cancer and can affect growth. It has been found to protect against a variety of serious, if common, conditions including arteriosclerosis, cancer, arthritis, cirrhosis and emphysema.

Selenium is incorporated by the body into one of its major defenses against attack, an antioxidant enzyme that places the mineral strategically at each of it active molecular sites. The "micronutrient" selenium is also active against excessive blood clotting, and in this way protects against coronary artery disease, heart attacks and stroke.

There are various theories about why and how we age. It is fascinating to note that no matter which of these theories we consider, selenium plays an essential part in countering the effects of aging. It certainly reduces the likelihood of developing many of the diseases associated with aging.

Scientists have studied the relationship between the level of selenium in the soil and the development of a variety of cancers. Their nearly incontestable conclusion: A high concentration of selenium corresponds to a low rate of these cancers, and a low rate of selenium corresponds to a high rate of cancers.

Venezuela, which has a high selenium content in its soils, has less than one quarter of the United States' mortality rate from cancer of the large intestine. In Japan, where selenium levels are high, the incidence of breast cancer is low. But when Japanese women move to the United States, their chances of developing breast cancer are just as high as women born here.

Studies from around the world confirm the relationship between adequate levels of serum selenium in the blood and resistance to many cancers. Other experiments suggest that selenium may also be effective against certain types of cancer tumors once they have developed.

On another front, increases in immune responses have been measured in test subjects given large doses of selenium. In experiments, this boost in immunity has been shown to be effective against malaria and, in animals, leptospirosis. In a study of AIDS patients, selenium levels were found to be subnormal, although it is not yet understood whether a deficiency of selenium contributes to the disease or if AIDS reduces selenium levels.

A swath of the southern United States crossing through Georgia and the Carolinas is known as the stroke belt. Not only does this region have the nation's highest stroke rate, it is also know for a very high incidence of heart disease. Not surprisingly, soils in this are very low in selenium. This supports the observation that cardiovascular disease increases as selenium absorption decreases. A similar situation has been found in Finland.

Toxic heavy metals such as mercury and cadmium, as well as alcohol, various drugs and cigarette smoke, can all be detoxified by selenium. It is thought the mineral combines with the toxins to yield inert compounds. Selenium may also be able to detoxify some types of carcinogenic fats.

Selenium has also been shown to contribute to the production of sperm and to sperm motility.

As an anti-inflammatory, selenium is an effective treatment for arthritis and other autoimmune diseases. It is used to treat a condition called Kashin-Beck disease, which affects the joints of millions of people in a region of China where the soil known to be deficient in soil selenium. In this use, it can be effective against growth retardation, joint enlargement, deformity of the spinal column and muscular atrophy, if given soon enough.

Chromium—Dietary Insulin!

Prior to the 1950s, chromium was thought to be nothing more than a toxic trace metal. Then, in an experiment with rats, it was discovered that feeding them brewer's yeast corrected glucose intolerance—an inability to remove sugar from the blood to nourish the cells–which is one of the characteristics of diabetes. Much work was conducted to isolate the specific component of the yeast responsible for this remarkable cure. It was finally discovered and called glucose tolerance factor (GTF).,

Chromium is available in whole grain cereals, black pepper, meat products and cheese—as well as in brewer's yeast.

A deficiency of chromium, besides leading to glucose intolerance, is know known to cause impaired growth, elevated blood cholesterol, fatty deposits in the arteries, decreased sperm count, in fertility plus an overall decrease in lifespan.

Marginal chromium deficiency is thought to be fairly common in the United States due to a diet of highly refined foods. Studies have also revealed a dramatic lifelong slide in the level of chromium present in the body tissues, accompanied by a slow rise in glucose intolerance. It is theorized that this process may contribute to aging.

We cannot live without glucose, but it must be very precisely regulated in the body. Too much can react adversely with many different biological molecules, including hemoglobin, proteins in membranes and possibly even DNA and RNA. Chromium is vital to the body's sensitivity to insulin, which in turn allows us to regulate the use of glucose.

Aging, pregnancy, consumption of refined foods, and even strenuous exercise can all contribute to the depletion of chromium in the body.

Hypoglycemic patients—those with dangerously low blood sugar levels—have experienced an increase in blood sugars after taking 200 micrograms of chromium daily.

Chromium may also be a part of the cardiovascular disease puzzle. Some researchers found that patients with coronary artery disease have significantly lower levels of chromium than healthy people. Others have reported supplements of chromium can decrease the overall level of cholesterol in the blood, while increasing the level of high density lipoproteins (HDLs). These are the cholesterols considered to prevent cardiovascular disease.

Molybdenum—Nutrition's Poison Control Center!

Rare in the crust of the earth we call home, molybdenum is equally rare in the human body. As a trace mineral, it is found in all tissues of the human body. Molybdenum is required for several key enzymes to function properly. Recently, science has come to understand more about molybdenum's role in the human body and have identified the deficiency symptoms. For example, a high rate of cancer of the esophagus in one area of China has been attributed to a lack of molybdenum.

Perhaps most fascinating of all, the extreme scarcity of molybdenum as a geologically occurring mineral and its widespread presence in living things has supported the theory that life was planted on earth by extraterrestrial sources.

Organ meats, grains, legumes, leafy vegetables, milk and beans are all good dietary sources of molybdenum.

In the body, molybdenum activates the enzyme sulfite oxidase, which acts to counteract the toxic effects of some of the hazardous substances we encounter daily. For example, this process is used to counter the poisonous effects of the sulfites that are used extensively as food preservatives. Without the molybdenum stimulated response to these poisons, we would experience nausea, diarrhea, acute asthma attacks, loss of consciousness, and even death. Additionally, the bisulfate form of this pollutant destroys vitamin B$_1$ unless it is preserved by molybdenum.

Uric acid—one of the body's most important scavengers of dangerous free radicals—is produced by another molybdenum activated enzyme. These toxic oxygen radicals are believed to be a major cause of degenerative disease and aging.

Bioflavonoids–Quercetin, Rutin, And Hesteperidin—The Hidden Protectors!

Widely available in the plants we eat, bioflavonoids are found in the leaves, flowers, and stems where they provide protection and color to the plants' tissues. Good sources for bioflavonoids include fruits (especially citrus fruits such as lemons), vegetables, nuts, seeds and buckwheat. Leaves, flowers and bark can also provide the substances when brewed as tea.

First popularized in human nutritional use decades ago as protectors of capillaries, the tiniest of our blood vessels, the bioflavonoids don't completely fit the definition of a vitamin, and no clear-cut deficiency symptoms have been recognized.

Medicines They Tried To Keep from You!

In 1968, spurred by an inconclusive study by the National Academy of Sciences and the National Research Council, the United States Food and Drug Administration declared bioflavonoids to be "ineffective for treating any human conditions whatsoever" and ordered them removed from the market as drugs. They have continued to be available to consumers as food supplements sold in health food stores.

But the government's bioflavonoid prohibition, perhaps encouraged by the pharmaceutical industry's interest in pushing nutrition OUT OF the margins of accepted health care, did little to reduce the public's interest in alternative—and vastly cheaper—forms of prevention and treatment. Now in demand because of the belief that vitamin C cannot work properly without them, bioflavonoid compounds are often found as a part of well-balanced multivitamin formulas.

And, in an interesting example of biological checks and balances, not only do we now believe that bioflavonoids are necessary for vitamin C to work in the body, it has been discovered that vitamin C itself protects the bioflavonoid quercetin from oxidation, enabling it to work!

Another Army Of Defenders At Your Disposal!

There is also convincing evidence that bioflavonoids themselves have antioxidant actions. By the 1980s, new studies were being published that suggested bioflavonoids had all sorts of previously unknown beneficial properties. A 1984 paper published in *Trends in Pharmacological Sciences* stated that bioflavonoids have "...potent anti-allergy, anti-inflammatory, and anti-viral activity."

During the Second International Conference on Antiviral Research, a number of researchers reported on anti-viral properties of the bioflavonoids. Derivatives of quercetin were found to be effective against a variety of viruses, including polio, ECHO, coxsackie virus and the rhinoviruses responsible for the common cold. It should come as no surprise that the researchers also discovered quercetin had no anti-viral properties by itself—it had to be used in conjuction with vitamin C!

Hesteperidin and quercetin have also been found to be active against herpes type 1, respiratory viruses and influenza viruses in the laboratory. Tests also suggest they have an effect on cells that cause allergic reactions, slowing the release of the histamines that cause sneezing, running noses and itchy, watering eyes.

Several classes of bioflavonoids have also been found to be anti-inflammatories and anti-spasmodic agents.

In recent years, there has been an increased interest in the medicinal properties of herbs. A number of investigators have pointed out that bioflavonoids appear to be the active ingredients in many herbs that have been in use as medicines since the dawn of time.

All of the vitamins, minerals, bioflavonoids and other nutrients mentioned in this chapter are commonly available in health food and vitamin stores.

25

Do Ulcers And Asthma Have A Common Connection—Water?

Often even the most diligent scientists forget the old sayings: "Simplicity is genius," and, "The answer is right in front of your nose!"

What we're about to tell you drew comments like "That's impossible!" and "That's hokey!" from scientists UNTIL THEY READ THE RESEARCH PAPERS!

Far back in medical history as well as today, doctors recommend that you drink six to eight glasses of water a day. You probably learned that in a grammar or high school health class.

Designer Waters Created A Great Health Trend!

The reason, doctors tell us, is that the water is needed to cleanse our body's systems and keep them operating properly!

Until a few years ago when it became a fad to drink "designer waters", rarely would you find a person who drank even six eight ounce glasses of water a day. Soda, coffee and tea don't count because they usually contain caffeine. Caffeine is a diuretic, which causes your body to loose water.

Unfortunately, medical science has done very little research on water until recently eventhough the body is made up of 75% water. The brain contains almost 85%.

Dr. F. Batmanghelidj, who graduated from the prestigious St. Mary's Medical School of London University, finally discovered the real value of water when he was doing research on stomach ulcers.

The stomach produces a very strong acid which is needed to break down the foods we eat into usable nutrients. The lining of the walls of the stomach is a mucus membrane which is usually unaffected by the acid.

All Ulcer Sufferers Are Dehydrated!

This acid is constantly being replaced. However, it is still very strong and cannot go into the intestines at full strength. So the pancreas produces a watery bicarbonate solution which neutralizes the acid and allows it to go into the intestines.

Dr. Batmanghelidj, while studying over 3000 patients with ulcers, discovered that ALL of them were suffering from dehydration.

He found that when the pancreas doesn't have enough water to neutralize the acid, it stimulates a muscle spasm of the sphincter muscle between the stomach and duodenum. The result is stomach pain!

Water Stops Ulcer Pain In 20 Minutes!

Dr. Batmanghelidj determined that when someone was having stomach pain, he could stop it within 20 minutes by having the patient drink three glasses of water.

As a daily regimen, the doctor urged all the ulcer patients in his research group to drink eight to ten glasses of water a day—and especially one a few minutes BEFORE each meal.

95% Cure Rate!

His research showed that over 95% of those who religiously followed his instruction no longer had ANY ulcer problems after three months.

Dr. Batmanghelidj suggests that you should reduce your ulcer medication by 10% a week for those 90 days until you are not using it at all.

For those who are technically oriented and want to examine his research, you'll find it in the 1983 edition of the *Journal of Clinical Gastroenterology.*

Why Don't Doctors Recommend This Treatment?

There are a few reasons: One, the lack of knowledge of these findings; two, disbelief without testing it; and three, the cynical profiteering doctors probably figure they will lose a customer which they would most likely have for a lifetime!

If you are suffering from ulcers, it doesn't cost anything to try it. But do it religiously, and stop drinking coffee, tea or soda that contains caffeine.

Asthma Relief Was A Side Effect!

A substantial number of the 3000 ulcer patients in the study had asthma. Many of them reported that their breathing problems had cleared up since they started drinking the water regularly.

This prompted Dr. Batmanghelidj to begin studying the effects of water on our breathing apparatus. He wasn't surprised when he found the reason for asthma was chronic dehydration.

Most Water Lost From Our Body Escapes As Breath!

When it is cold outside, you notice the steam that comes out of your lungs when you breathe. Of course, that's water vapor. Everytime you exhale, you release water—and even more in the summer, although it isn't visible.

Dr. Batmanghelidj found that when you don't have enough water in your system, the lung tissues constrict to reduce fluid loss.

What he discovered is revolutionary in medicine and not yet accepted, but here is how it works. Dr. Batmanghelidj discovered that the histamine in your lungs and bronchials tries to requisition water from other tissues. If the histamine can't get any water from the other tissues (most have water conservation mechanisms also), it keeps the lungs constricted.

If the histamine keeps the lungs constricted for long periods of time, chronic inflammation results. The bronchials also become inflamed and spasm.

Relieving The Symptom Not The Cause!

When you have this problem, doctors prescribe antihistamines, which suppress the body's need for water. They give temporary relief, but the cause of the problem remains.

Dr. Batmanghelidj says that the constant lack of water destroys cells in the lungs continually and therefore reduces its capability.

He presented his research on histamines and water deficiency at the Third Interscience World Conference On Inflammation, Antirheumatics and Analgesics in 1989 and astounded scientists from around the world.

Cured In A Matter Of Days!

Dr. Batmanghelidj has proven his theory works in literally hundreds of cases. Just like the ulcer problem, if you drink eight to ten glasses of water a day, the asthma will disappear and not return as long as you maintain the water regimen. Remember—no caffeine!

Nancy Drew-Jones, a member of our organization, overheard a staff member discussing the amazing findings of Dr. Batmanghelidj. Ms. Jones has suffered with asthma for over 10 years, and almost died a few years ago during a Stage Four attack!

"I wondered why my asthma symptoms had decreased so quickly and dramatically," she exclaimed. "I just started the Jenny Craig diet, which requires me to drink eight to ten glasses of water each day. Before, I wouldn't even walk across a room without bringing my nebulizer with me. Now I hardly ever use it, and it has been only a week since I started drinking that quantity of water." (A nebulizer turns a liquid bronchial dilating drug into a vapor which is sprayed into the throat.)

Cholesterol Count Lowered
With Only Water!

In Chapter 15 we explained the function of cholesterol in your body. Every cell uses cholesterol to hold it together and prevent various substances from entering or leaving the cell.

Dr. Batmanghelidj claims that when there is a water deficiency in the body, it produces more cholesterol to help prevent the loss of water from the cells. The blood cells are no different. However if the water deficiency is constant, he believes that is the reason excess cholesterol collects on the walls of veins.

There is no evidence that the doctor conducted a double blind study on the subject, but he claims that many of his patients have lowered high cholesterol levels substantially by drinking eight to ten glasses of water a day. Numerous patients lost weight also.

Are Diuretics Dangerous For
High Blood Pressure Sufferers?

Dr. Batmanghelidj says that when your body has a water deficiency it has to apply force to move water to the most needed area. That force or pressure is called hypertension. Therefore, high blood pressure is caused by dehydration.

Again the doctor is at odds with the medical establishment because they prescribe diuretics to alleviate high blood pressure. Diuretics accelerate the movement of water out of your body!

Most doctors say you have to reduce your salt intake when you have high blood pressure. Dr. Batmanghelidj claims that salt is important because it keeps more water in the tissues.

You'll Never Stop Taking
High Blood Pressure Drugs!

He also reports that hypertensives never get off drugs. First they get diuretics but their condition gets worse as a result. Then they receive a prescription for a beta blocker, then a calcium blocker and finally bypass surgery. Dr. Batmanghelidj says establishment doctors are slowly killing people who have high blood pressure.

From a scientific viewpoint, the doctor's theory does have substantial logic going for it eventhough it is 180 degrees from the establishment theories. The current treatment of high blood pressure is somewhat reminiscent of the 1700s when doctors thought "bad blood" was the cause of illness. So they bled people and used leeches to suck the blood from them. Most people died from the treatment.

Dr. Batmanghelidj says the American Medical Association (AMA) refused to even examine his research and theory. It appears the establishment still wants to suck blood out of patients with high priced drugs that make conditions worse and costly surgery that doesn't work.

The Proof Is In The Pudding!

It doesn't cost anything to try the water treatment. Dr. Batmanghelidj claims that he has hundreds of case histories of successfully lowering high blood pressure with water. Why not try it? It certainly can't hurt you.

A gentleman in our office who has mild high blood pressure tried taking 10 glasses of water a day. Within three days, his blood pressure was within a few points of normal and continued to be in the following weeks even as we wrote this chapter.

Water Helps Constipation!

Another side effect the doctor noticed in his studies was that people with chronic constipation often returned to normal—even after suffering for as much as thirty years with no relief.

Other Side Effects!

For most people, imbibing even six to eight eight ounce glasses of water a day will be a dramatic lifestyle change. The side effect you will probably experience is that you'll be urinating more often.

Dr. Batmanghelidj says that the amount of water you need is relative to your body size: six glasses for small people; eight for the average sized body and 10 to 12 for the large or obese person.

The doctor has written a fascinating book entitled, *Your Body's Many Cries For Water*, which contains many more important details about the foregoing plus information about other illnesses that can be alleviated with water. You can order the book from your local bookstore, or mail your order to Global Health Solutions, Dept. 1000, P.O.Box 3189, Falls Church, VA 22043. It is only $14.95 plus $3.00 shipping and handling.

A Built In Excuse!

If someday the medical establishment accepts Dr. Batmanghelidj's discoveries, they will have a handy excuse: "We've been preaching since modern medicine began that you need to drink six to eight glasses of water a day!"

Conclusion!

In marketing it is commonly known that "preventive" type products don't sell anywhere near to the volume of products that offer status, improved appearance, comfort, sensual enjoyment and entertainment.

But if you are sick, those things don't mean much. Feeling better and being healthy are your major concerns.

So then logic dictates that if you are to enjoy life, entertainment, travel, fine food, clothes, cars and be comfortable, you must be in good health. Even if you are wealthy and not healthy, you won't find much joy in life.

In Chapter 24, Dr. Cheraskin's research showed us that doctors, who took the most vitamins and minerals, were the healthiest with the least sickness. This certainly proved that "prevention is the best cure!"

However, that information is not worth anything unless you do something about it. Only you are responsible for your health. Don't wait until you get sick. That's like worrying about tooth decay after all your teeth have fallen out!

END

BIBLIOGRAPHY

Abe, N., Ebina, T. & Ishida, N. (1982). "Interferon induction by glycyrrhizin and glycyrrhetinic acid in mice." *Microbial Immunol.*, v. 26, pp. 535-539.

Abonyi, M., Kisfaludy, S. & Szalay, F. (1984) Therapeutic effect of (+)- cyanidanol-3 in toxic alcoholic liver disease and in chronic active hepatitis." *Acta Phsiol. Hung.*, 64, pp. 455-460

Adachi, K. & Sadai, M. (1985). "The hair growing product no. 82447." Japanese patent application.

Adachi, K. (1987). "Mechanism on hair growing effect of PDG." *Proceedings of the 17th World Congress of Dermatology.*

Ala El Din Barradah, M, Shoukry, I. & Hegazy, M. (1967). "Difrarel 100 in the treatment of retinal vascular disorders and high myopia." *Bulletin of the Opthamological Society of Egypt*, v. 60, p. 251.

Albert-Puleo, M. (1980). "Fennel and anise as estrogenic agents." *J. Ethnopharmacology,* v. 2, pp. 337-344.

Alfieri, R. & Sole, P. (1964). "Influences des anthocyanosides admistres par voie parenterale sur l'adaptoelectroretinogramme du lapin."*C.R. Soc. Biol.*v. 158, p. 2338.

Altman, L. (1992). "Prostrate drug's effects cited." *New York Times*, June 23. Ask-Upmark (1967). "Prostatitis and its treatment." *Acta Med. Scand.*, v. 181, pp. 355-357.

AMA Laboratories (1988) Independent unpublished cross-over, double blind study conduct ed by AMA Laboratories, of Tri-Genesis Hair Growth Formula.

Annin, P.; Underwood, A.; "A Week of Woes Raises More Questions About Saint Merck", *Newsweek,* Aug. 2, 1993.

Aslan, A. (1985). *Specifications Regarding the Technique and Action of Gerovital H3 Treatment After 34 Years of Usage.* Bucharest,Romania: Natl. Inst. of Ger.

Baetgen, D. (1961). "Results of the treatment of epidemic hepatitis in children with high doses of ascorbic acid." *Medizinische Monatschrift,* v. 15, pp. 30-36.

Bailliart, J.P. (1969). "Tentative d' amelioration de la vision nocturne." *Le Medicine de Reserve,* v. 121.

Baraona, E. & Lieber, C. (1979). "Effects of ethanol on lipid metabolism." *J. Lipid Res.,* v. 20, pp. 289-315.

Barker, H., Frank, O., Thind, I.C., et al. (1979). "Vitamin profiles in elderly persons living at home or in nursing homes versus profile in healthy young subjects." *J. Am. Geriatrics Society,* v. 10, pp. 444-450.

Barry, M. (1990). "Epidemiology and natural history of benign prostatic hyperplasia." *Urologic Clinics of N. America,* v. 17, no. 3, pp. 495-507.

Baur, H. & Staub, H. (1954). "Treatment of hepatitis with infusions of ascorbic acid: Comparison with other therapies." *Journal of the A.M.A.,* v. 156, p. 565.

Beattie, A., Campbell, B., Goldberg, A. & Moore, M. (1976). "Blood-lead and hypertension." *Lancet,* ii, pp. 1-3.

Beck, M. (1992). "Menopause." *Newsweek,* May 25.

Beisel, W.R. (1990). "Future role of micronutrients on immune functions." *Annal of the New York Acad. of Sciences,* v. 587, pp. 267-274.

Berengo, A. & Esposito, R. (1975) "A double-blind trail of (+)-cyanidanol-3 in viral hepatitis" *New Trends in the Therapy of Liver Diseases,* Springer-Verlang, Basel, pp. 1177-1181.

Bever. B. & Zahnd G.R. (1979). "Plants with oral hypoglycemic action." *Quarterly J. of Crude Drug Research* v. 17, pp. 139-196.

Birchall, J.D. & Espie, A.W. (1986). "Biological implications of the interaction of silicon with metal ions." *Ciba Foundation Symposium,* v. 121, p. 140.

Blondell, J.M. (1980). "The anticarcinogenic effect of magnesium." *Med. Hypotheses,* v. 6, pp. 863-871.

Blum, A., Doelle, W., Kortum, K., et al. (1977) "Treatment of acute viral hepatitis with (+)-cyanidanol-3" *Lancet,* ii, pp. 1153-1155.

Boari, C., Montanari, M., Galleti, G.P., et al. (1975). "Occupational toxic liver diseases. Therapeutic effects of silymarin" Min. Med., 72, pp. 2679-2688.

Boeryd, B. & Hallbgren, B. (1980). "The influence of the lipid composition of the feed given to mice on the immunocompetence and tumor resistance of the progeny." *Intl. J. of Cancer,* v. 26. pp. 241-246.

Bombardierei, G., Minalini, A., Bernardi, L. & Rossi, L. (1985). "Effects of s-adenosyl-l-methionine in the treatment of Gilbert's syndrome." *Curr,. Ther. Res.,* v. 37, pp. 580-585.

Boosalis, M.G., Evans, G.W. & McClain, C.J. (1983). "Impaired handling of orally administered zinc in pancreatic insufficiency." *Am. J. of Clin. Nutrition,* v. 37, pp. 268-271.

Bordia, A. & Bansal, H.C. (1973). "Essential

oil of garlic in prevention of atheroslcerosis." *The Lancet,* ii, p. 1491.

Boyd, E.M. & Berry, N.E. (1939). "Prostatic hypertrophy as part of a generalized metabolic disease. Evidence of the presence of a lipopenia." *J. of Urology,* v. 41, pp. 406-411.

Brattstrom, L.E., Hultberg, B.L. & Hardebo, J.E. (1985). "Folic acid responsive postmenopausal homocysteinemia." *Metabolism,* v. 34, pp. 1073-1077.

Brohult, A., Brohult, J., Brohult, S. & Joelsson, I. (1977). "Effect of alkyglycerols on the frequency of injuries following radiation therapy for carcinoma of the uterine cervix." *Acta Obstet. Gynecol. Scane.,* v. 56, no. 4, p. 441.

Bricklin, M. (1990). "The prostatic cancer group has swithched to a low-risk one." New York, NY: Penguin Books, pp. 438-439.

Canini, F., Bartolucci, A., Cristallini, E., et al (1985). "Use of Silymarin in the treatment of alcoholic hepatic stenosis" *Clin. Ther.,* 114, pp. 307-314.

Carlisle, E.M. (1986). "Silicon as an essential trace element in animal nutrition." *Ciba Foundation Symposium,* v. 121, p. 123.

Castleman, M. (1991). *The Healing Herbs.*

Catheart, R.F. (1981). "The method of determining proper doses of vitamin C for the treatment of disease titrating to bowel tolerance." *J. Orthmol. Psychiat.,* v. 10, pp. 125-132.

Cavalieri, S, (1974). "A controlled clinical trial of Legalon in 40 patients." *Gazz. Med. Ital.,* v. 133, pp. 628-635.

Champault, G., Patel, J.C. & Bonard, A.M. (1984). "A double-blind trial of an extract of the plant *Sereno repens* in benign prostatic hyperplasia." *Brit. J. Clin. Pharmacol.,* v. 18, pp. 461-462.

Chandra, R.K. (1987). "Nutrition and immunity: I. basic considerations. II. practical applications." *J. Dent. Child.,* v. 54, no. 3, pp. 193-197.

Chang, H.M. & But, P. [eds.] (1986). *Pharmacology and applications of Chinese Materia Medica.*

Cohen, L. & Litzes, R. (1981). "Infrared spectroscopy and magnesium content of bone mineral in osteoporotic women." *Isr. J. Med. Sci.,* v. 17, pp. 1123-1125.

Conn, H. (1981) [ed.] "International Workshop on (+)-Cyanidanol-3 in Diseases of the Liver" Royal Society of Medicine Symposia Series no. 47, Academic Press, London.

Cookson, F.B., Altshcul, R. & Federoff, S. (1967). "The effects of alfalfa on serum cholesterol and in modifying or preventing cholesterol induced atherosclerosis in rabbits." *J. of Atherosclerosis Res.,* v. 7, pp. 69-81.

Costello, C.H. & Lynn, E.V. (1950). "Estrogenic substances from plants: glycyrrhiza glabra." *J. of the Am. Pharm. Assc.,* v. 39, pp. 177-180.

Daly, J.M., Dudrick, S.J. & Copeland, E.M. (1978). "Effects of protein depletion and repletion on cell-mediated immunity in experimental animals." Ann. Surg., v. 188, no. 6, pp. 791-796.

De Froment, P. (1974). "Unsaponifiable substance from alfalfa for pharmaceuticals and cosmetic uses." French Patent 2,187,328.

Doheny, K. (1992). "New laser approach to prostate surgery." *Los Angeles Times,* Aug. 12.

Donsbach, K.W. (1989). *The Prostate.* Rosarito Beach, Mexico: Wholistic Publications.

Dreisbach, R.H. *Handbook of Poisoning,* 11th edition, pp. 80-83. Los Altos, CA: Lange Medical Publication.

Duke, J.A. (1985) "Handbook of Medicinal Herbs." Boca Raton, FL: CRC Press.

Ehrenpreis, S., Balagot, R.C., Comaty, J.E., & Myles, S.B., (1978). "Naloxone reversible analgesia in mice produced by D-phenylalanine and hydrocinamic acid, inhibitors of carboxypep-tidase A." *Advances in Pain Research and Therapy,* vol. 3.

Ellis, F., Holesch, S. & Ellis, J. (1972). *"Incidence of osteoporosis in vegetarians and omnivores."* Am. J. of Clin. Nutrition, v. 25, pp. 555-558.

Evans, G.W. (1980). "Normal and abnormal zinc absorption in man and animals: the tryptophan connection." *Nutrition Reviews,* v. 38, pp. 137-141.

Evans, G.W. & Johnson, E.C. (1981). "Effect of iron, vitamin B-6 and picolinic acid on zinc absorption in the rat." *J. of Nutrition,* v. 111, pp. 68-75.

Evans, Wm.; Rosenberg, I.H.; BIOMARKERS, 1991, Simon & Shuster.

Faber, K. (1958) "The dandelion – Taraxacum officinale Weber" *Pharmazie,* 13, pp. 423-435.

Fahim, W.S., Harman, J.M. Clevenger, T.H., et. al. (1982). "Effect of panax ginseng on testosterone level and prostate in male rats," *Arch. Androl.*

Feinblatt, H.M. and Gant, J.C. (1958). "Palliative treatment of benign prostatic hypertrophy: value of glycine, alanine, glutamic acid combination." *J. of the Maine Med. Assc.*

Felter, H.W. (1983) *The Eclectic Materia Medica, Pharmacology and Therapeutics.* Portland, OR: Eclectic Medical Publication.

Fisher, J.A. (1990). *The Chromium Program.* New York: Harper & Row.

Folkers, K. Watanabe, T. & Kaji, M. (1977). "Critique of coenzyme Q10 in biochemical research on cardiovascular disease." *J. Mol. Med.,* v. 2, pp. 461-460.

Folkers, K. & Yamamura, Y. (eds.) (1984) *Biomedical and Clinical Aspects of Coenzyme Q,* v. 4. Amsterdam: Elsevier Science Publishers.

Formann, S., Hashell, W. Vranizan, K., *et al.,* (1983). " The association of blood pressure and dietary alcohol: difference by age, sex and estrogen use." *Am. J. Epid.,* v. 118, pp. 497-507.

Francis, R.M. & Beaumont, D.M. (1987). "Involutional osteoporosis." Letter to the Editor. *New Eng. J. of Med.,* v. 316, p. 216.

Freudenheim, M. (1992). "Prostate treatment could be bonanza." *New York Times,* June 22.

Frezza, M., Possato, G., Chiesa, L., *et al* (1984). "Reversal of intrahepatic cholestasis of pregnancy in women after high dose s-adenosyl-l-methionine (SAMe) administration." *Hepatology,* v. 4, pp. 274-278.

Fujimoto, I., Hanai, A. & Oshima, A. (1979). "Descriptive epidemiology of cancer in Japan: current cancer incidence and survival data." *Natl. Cancer Ins. Monographs,* v. 53, pp. 5-15.

Gestetner, B., Assa, Y. Henis, Y., Birk, Y. & Bondi, A. (1971). Lucerne saponins. IV. Relation between their chemical constitution and hemolytic and anti-fungal activities." *J. of Science, Food and Agriculture,* v. 22, no. 4, pp. 168-172.

Gibbs, O.S. (1947). "On the curious pharmacology of hydrastis." *Fed. of Am. Soc. for Exp. Biol. Fed. Proc.,* v. 6, no. 1, p. 332.

Gilbert, A. & Carnot, P. (1896). "Note prelinair sur l'opotherapie hepatique." *Compt. Rend. Soc. Biol.,* v. 48, pp. 934-937.

Gil Del Rio, E. (1968). "Los antocianosidos del *Vaccinum myrtillus* en optalmologia." Gaz. Med de France, v. 18, June 25.

Gladwell, Malcolm; "Serious Side Effects Linked To Many Approved Drugs", *Wash. Post,* May 28, 1990.

Glauser, S., Bello, S. & Gauser, E. (1976). "Blood-cadmium levels in untreated hypertensive humans." *Lancet,* i, pp. 717-718.

Gorman, C.; "Can Drug Firms Be Trusted", *Time Mag.,* Feb, 10, 1992.

Goldin, B.R. & Gorbach, S.L. (1984). "The effect of milk and lactobacillus feeding on human intestinal bacterial enzyme activity." *Am. J. of Clin. Nutrition,* v. 39, pp. 756-761.

Goldstein, A.; 1992, "Overmedication Poses Significant Health Risk," *Wash. Post.*

Graber, C.D., Goust, M.M., Glassman, A.D., Kendall, R. & Loadholt, C.B. (1981). "Immunomodulating properties of dimethylglycine in humans." *J. of Infectious Diseases,* v. 143, no. 1, pp. 101-105.

Greenberg, J.; 1993, "Your Money Or Your Life", *Playboy.*

Grossman, M., Kirsner, J. & Gillespie, I. (1963). "Basal and histalog-stimulated gastric secretion in control subjects and in patients with peptic ulcer or gastric cancer." *Gastroenterology,* v. 45, pp. 14-26

Gruchow, H.W., Sobocinski, M.S. & Barboriak, J.J. (1985). "Alcohol, nutrient intake, and hypertension in U.S. adults." *J. of the A.M.A.,* v. 253, pp. 1567-1570.

Gutfeld, R.; 1993, "F.D.A. Attacks Drug Makers' Ads To Doctors", *Wall St. J.*

Habib, F.K., et al. (1976). "Metal-androgen interrelationships in carcinoma and hyperplasia of the human prostate." *J. Endocrinol.,* v. 71, no. 1, pp. 133-141.

Harman, D. (1981). "The aging process." *proceedings of the Nat. Acad. of Sciences,* v. 78, no. 11. pp. 7124-7128, November.

Hartroft, W.S., Porta, E.A. & Suzuki, M. (1964). "Effects of choline chloride on hepatic lipids after acute ethanol intoxication." *Q.J. Stuc. Alcohol,* v. 25, pp. 427-434.

Hasegaw, T. [ed.] (1975). *Proc. First Intersectional Cong. Int. Assoc. Microbiol. Soc.,* vol. 3, Tokyo University Press, pp. 432-442.

Havsteen, B. (1983) . "Flavonoids, a class of natural products of high pharmacological potency." *Biochem. Pharm.,* v. 32, no. 7, pp. 1141-1148.

Hikino, H., Kiso, Y., Wagner, H. & Fiebig, M. (1984). "Antihepatotoxic actions of flavonolignans from *Silybum marianum* fruits" *Planta Medica,* 50, pp. 248-250.

Hirayama, S., Kishikawa, H., Kume, T. & Tada, H. (1978). "Therapeutic effect of liver hydrolysate on experimental liver cirrhosis." *Nisshin Igaku,* v. 45, pp. 528-533.

Hochschild, R. (1973). "Effect of dimethylaminoethanol on the life span of senile male A/J mice." *Exp. Ger.,* pp. 185-191, v. 8.

Hodges, R. & Rebello, T. (1983). "Carbohydrates and blood pressure." *Ann. Int. Med.,* v. 98, pp. 838-814.

Hoffmann, D. (1991), *The New Holistic Herbal.* Rockport, MA: Element, Inc., pp. 69-70.

Holl, M.G. & Allen, L.H. (1988). "Comparative effects of meals high in protein, sucrose, or starch on human mineral metabolism and insulin secretion." *Am. J. of Clin. Nutrition,* v. 48, p. 1219.

Honegger, C. & Honegger, R. (1959). "Occurrence and quantitative determination of 2-dimethylaminoethanol in animal tissue extracts." *Nature,* pp. 550-552, v. 184.

Horton, R. (1984). "Benign prostatic hyperplasia: a disorder of androgen metabolism in the male." *J. of the Am. Ger. Soc.,* v. 32, pp. 380-385.

Hosein, E.A. & Bexton, B. "Protective action of carnitine on liver lipid metabolism after ethanol administration to rats." *Biochem. Pharm.,* v. 24, pp. 1859-1863.

Hunt, G.L. (1987). "Coenzyme Q10: Miracle Nutrient?" *Omni,* p. 24, Feb.

Hvalik, R., Hubert, H., Fabsitz, R. & Feinleib, M. (1983). "Weight and hypertension." *Ann. Int. Med.,* v. 98, pp. 855-859.

Hypertension Detection and Follow-Up Program Cooperative Group. (1977). "Race, education and prevalence of hypertension. *Am. J. of Epidemiology,* v. 106, pp. 351-361.

Infante-Rivard, C., Krieger, M., Gascon-Barre, M. & Rivard, G.E. (1986). "Folate deficiency among institutionalized elderly, public health impact." *J. Am. Ger. Soc.,* v. 34, pp. 311-214.

The Institute for Advanced Study of Human Sexuality Research Department (IASHSRD), 1990, *The* Avena sativa *Project: A Research Report on Sexual Health Care Products with Extract of* Avena sativa. San Francisco, CA.

Intelli-Scope (1992). "Natural Fat-loss," October, 1992, vol. 5.

Jameson, P.G. (1988). *The Herbal Handbook,* London: Brighton Press.

Jayle, G.E., Aubry, M., Gavini, M. & Braccini, G. (1965). "Etude concernant l' action sur la vision nocturne des anthocyanosides extraits de *Vaccinum myrtillus.*" Ann. Ocul., v. 198, p. 556.

1988 Joint National Committe. A report on detection, evaluation and treatment of high blood pressure. Arch. of Int. Med., v. 148, pp. 36-39.

Judd, A.M., MacLeod, R.M. and Login , I.S. (1984). "Zinc acutely, selectively and reversibly inhibits pituitary prolactin secretion." *Brain Research.,* v. 294, pp. 191-192.

Kagawa, T. (1978) "Impact of westernization on the Japanese. Changes in physique, cancer and logevity." *Prev. Med.,* v. 7, pp. 205-217.

Kamanna, V.S. & Chandrasekhara, N. (1982). "Effect of garlic on serum lipoproteins and lipprotein cholesterol levels in albino rats rendered hypercholesteremic by feeding cholesterol." *Lipids,* v. 17, no. 7, pp. 483-488.

Kamen, B. (1989). *Startling New Facts About Osteoporosis.* Novato, CA: Nutrition Encounter, Inc.

Kaplan, N.M. (1985). "Non-drug treatment of hypertension." *Ann. of Int. Med.,* v. 102, pp. 359-373.

Kershbaum, A., Pappajohn, D., Bellet, S., (1968). "Effect of smoking and nicotine on adrenocortical secretion." *J. of the A.M.A.,* v. 203, pp. 113-116.

Khaw, K.T. & Barrett-Connor, S. (1984). "Dietary potassium and blood pressure in a population." *Am. J. Clin. Nurt.,* v. 39, pp. 963-968.

Kinsella, K.G. (992). "Changes in life expectancy 1900-1990." Am. J. of Clin. Nutr., v. 55, pp. 1196S-1202S.

Kiso, Y., Suzuki, Y., Watanabe, N., *et al.* (1983). "Antihepatotoxic principles of *curcumba longa* rhizomes." *Planta Medica,* v. 49, pp. 185-187.

Klenner, F.R. (1971). "Observations on the administration of ascorbic acid when employed beyond the range of a vitamin in human pathology." *J. Applied Nutr.,* v. 23, pp. 61-88.

Knodell, R.G., et al. (1981). "Vitamin C prohylaxis for post-transfusion hepatitis: lack of an effect in a controlled trial.: *Am. J. of Clin. Nutr.,* v. 34, p. 20.

Kotulak, R. & Gorner, R. (1991). "Science begins to reset the clock: new insights guide research into living younger, longer." *Chicago Tribune,* Dec. 8.

Krasinski, S.D., Russell, R.M., Furie, B.C., *et al* (1985). "The prevalence of vitamin K deficiency in chronic gastrointestinal disorders." *Am. J. of Clin. Nutr.,* v. 41, pp. 639-643.

Krieger, I., Cash, R. & Evans, G.W. (1984). "Picolinic acid in acrodermatitis enteropathica: evidence or a disorder of tryptophan metabolism." J. of Ped. Gastr. and Nutr., v. 3, pp. 62-68.

Kritchevsky, D. (1975). "Effect of garlic oil on experimental atherosclerosis in rabbits." *Artery,* v. 1, no. 4, pp. 319-323.

Kuagai, A., Nanboshi, M., Asanuma, Y., *et al.* (1967). "Effects of *glycyrrhizin* on thymolytic and immunosuppressive action of cortisone." *Endocrinol Japan,* v. 145, pp. 39-42.

Kugler, H. (1989). "Tyrosine's effect on the depression syndrome." *Prev. Med. Up-Date,* v. 2, no. 6.

Kugler, H. (1990a). "Procaine versus the DMAE-PABA formula." *Prev. Med. Up-Date,* v. 4, no. 11.

Lahtonen, R. (1985). "Zinc and cadmium concentrations in whole tissue and in separated epithelium and stroma from human benign prostatic hypertrophic glands." *Prostate,* v. 6, pp. 177-183.

Lancet (1986). "Citrate for calcium nephrolithiasis," p. 955.

Lang, T., Degoulet, P., Aime, F., et al. (1983) "Relationship between coffee drinking and blood pressure: analysis of 6,321 subjects in Paris." *Am. J. Card.,* v. 52, pp. 1238-1242.

Leake, A., Chisholm, G.D. & Habib, F.K. (1984a). "The effect of zinc on the 5-alpha-reduction of testosterone by the hyperplastic human prostate gland." *J. Steroid Biochem.,* v. 20, pp. 651-655.

Leake, A., Chisholm, G.D., Busuttil, A. and Habib, F.K. (1984a). "Subcellular distribution of zinc in the benign and malignant human prostate: evidence for a direct zinc androgen interaction." *Acta Endocrinology,* v. 105, pp. 281-288.

Leary, Warren E.; "Companies Accused of Overcharging For Drugs Developed With U.S. Aid", *N.Y. Times,* Jan. 20, 1993.

Lesourd, B.M. (1990). "Immunologic aging. Effect on denutrition." *Ann. Biol. Clin.,* v. 48, no. 5, pp. 309-318.

Leung, A.Y. (1980). *Ency. of Common Natural Ingredients Used in Food, Drugs, and Cosmetics.* New York, NY: John Wiley & Sons.

Levenson (1983). *J. Parenteral & Enteral Nutr.,* v. 7, no. 2, p. 181-183.

Lewis, A. (1990) *Dimethylaminoethanol (DMAE): An Overview of its Health Effects and Potential Uses.* Belmont Chemicals, Inc.

Lewis, H.L. & Memory P.F. *Medical Botany: Plant's Affecting Man's Health,* p. 401. New York: John Wiley & Sons.

Lewis, N.M. (1989). "Calcium supplements and milk: effects on acid-base balance and on retention of calcium, magnesium, and phosphorous." *Am. J. of Clin. Nutr.,* v. 49, p. 527.

Lippman, R. (1980). "Chemiluminescent measurement of free radicals and antioxidant molecular-protection inside living rat mitochondria." *Exp. Ger.,* v. 15, pp. 339-351.

Lucas, R.M. (1991). *Miracle Medicinal Herbs,* p. 6.

Malinow, M.R., McLaughlin, P. & Papworth, L. (1976). "Hypocholesterolemic effect of alfalfa in cholesterol-fed monkeys." *Intl. Symp. on Atherosclerosis,* Tokyo, Japan.

Mandell, M. (1985). *Lifetime Arthritis Relief System,* Berkeley Books.

Maros, T., Racz, G., Katonaj, B. & Kovacs, V. (1966, 1968). "The effects of *cynara scolymus* extracts on the regeneration of the rat liver." Arzneim-Forsch, 1966, v. 16, pp. 127-129: 1968, v. 18, pp. 884-886.

Marsh, A., Sanchez, T., Chaffee, F., et al. (1983). "Bone mineral mass in adult lacto-ovo-vegetarian and omnivorous adults." *Am. J. of Clin. Nutr.,* v. 37, pp. 453-456.

Martin, D., Mayes, P. & Rodwell, V. (1983). *Harper's Rev. of Biochem.* Los Altos, CA: Lange.

Masquelier, J. (1980). "Natural Products as Medicinal Agents. *J. of Nat. Products,* July.

Masquelier, J. (1987). "U.S. Patent No. 4,698,360," Oct. 6.

Matson, F., Grudy, S. & Crouse, J. (1982). *The Am. J. of Clin. Nutr.,* v. 35, pp. 697-700.

Maugh, T.H., II, (1992). "Scientists draw back veil on the mystery of aging." *Los Angeles Times,* Feb. 8.

Maynard, G., Franch, J.P. & Dorne, P.A. (1970). "Use of tetrahydroxy flaven diol in opthamology, in particular in diabetic retinopathies (based on 40 cases)." *Lyon Medical,* no. 4, Jan. 25.

McCaslin, F.E., Jr. & Janes, J.M. (1959). "The effect of strontium lactate in the treatment of osteoporosis." *Proc. Staff Meetings Mayo Clinic,* v. 34, p. 329.

Meneely, G. & Battarbee, H. (1976). "High sodium-low potassium environment and hypertension." *Am. J. Card.,* v. 38, pp. 768-781.

Meydani, S.N., Furukawa, T., Meydani M. & Blumberg, J.B. (1990). "Beneficial effect of dietary antioxidants on the aging immune system." Nutr. Immun. and Tox. Lab., USDA Human Nutr. Res. Center of Aging, Tufts Univ.

Middleton. E. (1984). "The flavonoids." *TIPS,* August 1984.

Milkie, G. (1972). "Diet and its effect on the visual system," presented at the Annual Meeting of the Am. Acad. of Optometry, New York, NY, Dec. 19.

Miller, E. (1974). "Deanol in treatment of levodopa-induced dyskinesias." Neurology, pp. 116-119, v. 24.

Miller, J.Z., Nance, W.E., Norton, J.A., Wolen, R.L., Griffith, R.S., Rose, R.J. (1977). "Therapeutic effect of vitamin C, a co-twin control study." J. of the A.M.A., v. 237, pp. 248-251.

Mindell, E. (1991) *Vitamin Bible,* pp. 64-65. New York: Warner Books.

Mitscher, L., Park, Y. & Clark, D. (1980). "Antimicrobial agents from higher plants: antimicrobial isoflavonoids from *glycyrrhiza glabra L. var. typica*." *J. Nat. Products,* v. 43, pp. 259-269.

Montgomery, R., Dryer, R., Conway, T. & Spector, A. (1980). "Biochemistry: a case-oriented approach." St. Louis, MO: Mosby.

Montini, M., Levoni, P., Angoro, A. & Pagani, G. (1975). "Controlled trial of cynarin in the treatment of the hyperlipemic syndrome." *Arzneim-Forsch,* v. 25, pp. 1311-1314.

Morales, A., Condra, M., Owen, J.A., Surridge, D.H., Fenemore, J. & Harris, C. (1987). "Is yohimbine effective in the treatment of organic impotence? Results of a controlled trial." *J. of Urol.,* pp. 1168-1172, v. 137, no. 6.

Morris, D.L.; "Squeeze On Pharmaceuticals", *Chem. Wk.,* Aug. 12, 1992.

Mowrey, D. (1986). *The Scientific Validation of Herbal Medicine.* New Canaan, CT: Keats Publishing.

Murata, A. (1975). "Viricidal activity of vitamin C: vitamin C for prevention and treatment of viral diseases" in Hasegawa, T. [ed.]. *Proc. First Intersectional Cong. Int. Assoc. Microbiol. Soc.,* v. 3, pp. 432-442. Tokyo Univ. Press.

Murav'ev, I.A. & Kononikhina, N.F. (1972). "Estrogenic properties of *glycyrrhiza glabra.*" *Rastitel'nye Resursy,* v. 8, no. 4. pp. 490-497.

Murphree, H., Pfeiffer, C. & Backerman, I. (1959). "The stimulant effect of 2-dimethyl-laminoethanol (deanol) in human volunteer subjects." *Clin. Phar. and Ther.,* pp. 303-310, v. 1, n. 3.

Nagai, K. (1970). "A study of the excretory mechanism of the liver–effect of liver hydrolysate on BSP excretion." *Jap. J. Gastroenterol.,* v. 67, pp. 633-638.

Nandkarni, A.K. (1954). *Indian Materia Medica.* Panvel 1954, v. 1., 3rd ed., pp. 189-190.

National Institutes of Health Consensus Conference: Osteoporosis (1984). J. of the A.M.A., v. 252, p. 799

Nicar, M.J. & Pak, C.Y.C. (1985). "Calcium bioavailability from calcium carbonate and calcium citrate." J. of Clin. Endo. and Metab., v. 61, pp. 391-393.

Nielsen, F.H. (1988). "Boron–an overlooked element of potential nutrition importance." *Nutrition Today,* Jan./Feb., pp. 4-7.

Nishinlhon J. of Derm. (1986). "LKF–a research team, clinical evaluation of LKF-A on male pattern alopecia," (pp. 738-748), v. 48, no. 4.

Nomura, A., Henderson, B.E. & Lee, J. (1978). "Breast cancer and diet among the Japanese in Hawaii." *Am. J. of Clin. Nutr.,* v. 31, pp. 2020-2025.

Nutrition Rev. (1984). "The function of the vitamin K-dependent proteins, bone GLA protein (BGP) and kidney GLA proteins (KGP)." V. 42, pp. 230-233.

Oba, K. (1986). "Development of hair growing product especially with a property of PDG." *Fragrance Journal* (pp. 109-114), v. 14, no. 5.

Ohbayashi, A., Akoka, T. & Tasaki, H. (1972). "A study of effects of liver hydrolysate on hepatic circulation." *J. Therapy,* v. 54, pp. 1582-1585.

Osvaldo, R. (1974). "2-dimethylaminoethanol (deanol): a brief review of its clinical efficacy and postulated mechnism of action." *Curr. Ther. Res.,* pp. 1238-1242, v. 16, n. 11.

Padova, C., Tritapepe, R., Padova, F. *et al.* (1984). "S-adenosyl-L-methionine antagonizes oral contraceptive-induced bile cholesterol supersaturation in healthy women: preliminary report of a controlled randomized trial." *Am. J. Gastroenterol.,* v. 79, pp. 941-944.

Paganelli, G.M., Biasco, G., Brandi, G., (1992). "Effect of vitamin A, C, and E supplementation on rectal cell proliferation in patients with colorectal adenomas." *J. of the Nat. Can. Inst.,* v. 84, no. 1, p. 4751.

Par A., Horvath, T., Bero, T., *et al.* (1984) "Inhibition of hepatic drug metabolism by (+)-cyanidanol-3 (catergen) in chronic alcoholic liver disease" *Acta Physiol. Hung.,* v. 54, pp. 449-454.

Passwater, R.A. (1987) . "Coenzyme Q-10: The Nutrient of the 90's " *Whole Foods,* pp. 9-13, April.

Passwater (1991). *The New Supernutrition.* New York: Pocket Books.

Pauling, L. (1986). *How To Live Longer and Feel Better.* New York: Avon Books.

Pautler, E.L., Mega, J.A. & Tengerdy, C. "A pharmacologically potent natural product in the bovine retina."

Pelletier, O. (1968). "Smoking and vitamin C levels in humans." *Am. J. Clin. Nutri.,* v. 21, pp. 1254-1258.

Pelton, R. & Pelton, T.C. (1989). *Mind Food & Smart Pills.* New York: Doubleday.

Peltz, James F.; 1992, "Insurer To Reimburse Cost of Non-Surgical Heart Care.", *L.A. Times.*

Penn, N.D. *et al.* (1990). "The effect of dietary supplementation with vitamins A, C and E on cell-mediated immune function in elderly long-stay patients." *Age and Aging* v. 20, no. 20, pp. 169-174.

Peretz, A.M., *et al.* (1990). "Enhancement of the immune response by selenium: clinical trials." *Artzl. Lab.,* v. 36, pp. 299-304.

Petersdorf, R. (1983). *Harrison's Princ. of Int. Med.* New York, NY: McGraw-Hill.

Piazza, M., Guadagnino, V., Picciotto, J., et al. (1983). "Effect of (+)- cyanidanol-3 in acute HAV, HBV, and non-A, non-B viral hepatitius." *Hepatology,* v. 3, pp. 45-49.

Pierkle, J.L., Scwartz, J. Landis, J.R. & Harlan, W.R. (1985). "The relationship between blood lead levels and blood pressure and its cardiovascular risk implications." *Am. J. Epid.,* v. 121, pp. 246-258.

Pizzorno, J.E. & Murray, M.T. (1988). *A Textbook of Nat. Med.,* ch. IV "Hepatoprotection." John Bastyr College Publications.

Pointet-Guillot, U. (1958). "Contribution a l'etude chimique et pharmacologique de la reglisse." These, Paris.

Pompeii, R., Pani, A., Flore, O., Marcialis, M. & Loddo, B. (1980) "Antiviral activity of glycyrrhizic acid." *Experientia,* v. 36, pp. 304-305.

Potter, J.F. & Beevers D.G. (1984). "Pressor effect of alcohol in hypertension." *Lancet,* pp. 119-121.

Poydock, M.E., et al., (1979). "Inhibiting effect

368

of vitamins C and B-12 on the mitotic activity of ascites tumors." *Exp. Cell. Biol.,* vol. 47, no. 3. pp. 210-217.

Pristautz, H. (1975). "Cynarin in the modern treatment of hyperlipemias." *Wiener Medizinische Wocheschrift,* v. 1223, pp. 705-709.

Ralz, G.; "Drug Companies' Profit Margins Top Most Industries...", *Wall St. J.,* Feb. 26, 1993.

Ramesha A., Rao N., Rao A.R., *et al.* (1990). "Chemoprevention of 7, 12 dimethyl-benz[a]anthracene-induced mammary carcinogensis in rat by the combined actions of selenium, magensium, ascorbic acid, and reintylacetate." *Jap. J. of Can. Res.,* v. 81, pp. 1239-1246.

Rao, C., Rao, V. & Steinman, B. (1981). "Influence of bioflavonoids on the metabolism and crosslinking of collagen." *Ital. J. Biochem.,* v. 30, pp. 259-270.

Reap, E.A. & Lawson, J.W. (1990). "Stimulation of the immune response by dimethylglycine, a nontoxic metabolite." *J. Lab. Clin. Med.,* v. 115, pp. 481-486.

Recker, R.R. (1985). "The effect of milk supplements on calcium metabolism and calcium balance." *Am. J. of Clin. Nutri.,* v. 41, p. 254.

Regenstein, L. (1982). *America the Poisoned.* Washington, D.C.: Acropolis.

Reid, K., Surridge, D.H. Morales, A., Condra, M. Harris, C., Owen, J. & Fenemore, J. (1987). "Double-blind trial of yohimbine in treatment of psychogenic impotence." *Lancet,* v. 2, no. 8556, pp. 421-423.

Robertson, J., Donner, A & Trevithick, J. (1991). "A possible role for vitamins C and E in cataract prevention." Am. J. of Clin. Nutri., v. 53, pp. 346-351.

Robbins, S., Cotran, R. & Kuman, V. (1984). *Pathologic Basis of Disease.* Philadelphia, PA: W.B. Saunders.

Rogers, L.L. & Pelton, R.B. (1957). "Effect of glutamate on IQ scores of mentally deficient children." *Tex. Rep. on Bio. and Children,* (pp. 84-90), v. 15, no. 1.

Rubenstein, E. & Federman, D.D. (1988). "Scientific American medicine." *Scien. Am.,* pp. 4:VII:1-6.

Rubin, R.; Hawkins, D; Poodolsky, D.; "A Double Dose Of Medicine", *U.S. News & World Rep.,* July 19, 1993.

Rundle, R.L.; Stevens, A.; "Investigators Intensify Crackdown On Fraud In The Health Industry", *Wall St. J.,* Aug. 16, 1993.

Sachan, D.A. & Rhew, T.H. (1983). "Lipotropic effect of carnitine on alcohol-induced hepatic stenosis." *Nutri. Rep. Int.,* v. 27, pp. 1221-1226.

Sachan, D.S., Rhew, T.H. & Ruark, R.A. (1984).

"Ameliorating effects of carnitine and its precursors on alcohol-induced fatty liver." *Am. J. of Clin. Nutr.,* v. 39, pp. 738-744.

Sadai, M. (1987). "Effect of PDG on cultured dermal papilla cells, especially with reference to ATP production and DNA synthesis." Presented at the *17th World Congress of Dermatology.*

Salmi, H.A. & Sarna, S. (1982). "Effects of silymarin on chemical, functional and morphological alteration of the liver. A double-blind controlled study." *Scand. J. Gastroenterol.,* 17, pp. 417-421.

Sanbe, K., Murata, T., Fujisawa, K. et al. (1973). "Treatment of liver disease–with particular reference to liver hydrolysates." *Jap. J. Clin, Exp. Med.,* v. 50, pp. 2665-2676.

Santillo, H. (1991). *Natural Healing with Herbs.*

Sarre, H. (1971) "Experience in the treatment of chronic hepatopathies with silymarin." *Arzeim-Forsch.,* 21, pp. 1209-1212.

Scheiber V. & Wohlzogen, F.X. (1978) "Analysis of a certain type of 2 X 3 tables, exemplified by biopsy findings in a controlled clinical trial." *Int. Clin. Pharmacol.,* v. 16, pp. 533-535.

Schomerus H., Wieman, K., Dolle, W. et al. (1984) "(+)-cyanidanol-3 in the treatment of acute viral hepatitis: a randomized controlled trial." *Hepatology,* v. 4, pp. 331-335.

Scott, W.W. (1945). "The lipids of the prostatic fluid, seminal plasma and enlarged prostate gland of man." *J. of Uro.,* v. 53, pp. 712-718.

Sharaf, A., Gomaa, N., El-Camal, M.H.A. (1975). "*Glycyrrhetic* acid as an active estrogenic substance separated from *glycyrrihiza glabra* (licorice)." *Egyp. J. of Pharm. Science,* v. 16, no. 2, pp. 245-251.

Sinquin, G., Morfin, R.F., Charles, J.F. & Floch, H.H. "Testosterone metabolism by homogenates of human prostates with benign hyperplasia: effects of zinc, cadmium, and other bivalent cations." *J. Steroid Biochem.,* v. 20, pp. 733-780.

Skrabal, F. Aubock, J. & Hortnagl, H. (1981). "Low sodium/high potassium diet for prevention of hypertension: probable mechanisms of action." *Lancet,* ii., pp. 895-900.

Smith-Barbaro, P., Hanson, D. & Reddy, B.S. (1981). "Carcinogen binding to various types of dietary fiber." *J. of the Nat Canc. Inst.,* v. 67, no. 2, pp. 495-497.

Stanko, R.T., Mendelow, H., Shinozuka, H. & Adibi, S.A. (1978). "Prevention of alcohol-induced fatty liver by natural metabolites and riboflavin." *J. Lab. Clin. Med.,* v. 91, pp. 228-235.

Stark, P.; "Not All Drug Lords Are Outlaws", *New York Times,* August 12, 1992.

369

Stolberg, S. (1992). "Rewiring the mind and body." *Los Angeles Times,* Nov. 30.

Stone, Leonard; "F.D.A. Seeks Labeling That Would List Side Effects Of Drugs On Elderly", *N.Y. Times,* 1992.

Surgeon General's Report on Nutrition and Health (1988). Washington, D.C.: U.S. Dept. of Health and Human Serv.

Susset, J.G., Tessier, C.D., Wincze, J., Bansal, S., Malhotra, & Schwacha, M.G. (1989). "Effect of yohimbine hydrochloride on erectile impotence: a double-blind study." *J. of Uro.,* pp. 1360-1363, v. 141, no. 6.

Suzuki H., et al. (1986) "Cianidanol therapy for HBe-antigen-positive chronic hepatitis: a multicenter, double-blind study." *Liver,* v. 6, p. 35.

Sydenstricker, V.P., et al. (1940). "Observations on the 'egg white' injury in man." *J. of the A.M.A.,* v. 118, pp. 1199-1200.

Theodoropoulos, G., Dinos, A., Dimitriou, P. & Archimandritis, A. (1981) "Effect of (+)-cyanidanol-3 in acute hepatitus" in Conn, H. [ed], Int. Workshop on (+)-cyanidanol-3 in Diseases of the Liver." *Roy. Soc. of Med. Intl. Symp. Series,* no. 47, Academic Press, London.

Thom, J., Morris, J., Bishop, A. & Blacklock, J.J. (1978). "The influence of refined carbohydrate on urinary calcium excretion." *Brit. J. of Uro.,* v. 50, pp. 459-464.

Thompson, J.S., Robbins, J. & Cooper, J.K. (1987). "Nutrition and immune function in the geriatric population." *Clinic. Geriatr. Med.,* v. 3, no. 2, pp. 309-317.

Thottam, J.; 1992 "Generic Drug Makers Prepare For Next Battle", *Wall St. J.*

Toufexis, A. (1992). "The new scoop on vitamins." *Time* magazine, pp. 54-59, April 6.

Tregarten, S.; "Prescription To Stop Drug Companies' Profiteering", *Wall St. J.,* Mar. 5, 1992.

Tsung and Hsu (1986). Yamada, Cyong, *et al.*

Tyihak, E. & Szende, B. (1970). "Basic plant proteins with antitumor activity." Hungarian Patent 798.

Tyroler, H.A., Heyden, S. & Hames, C.G. (1975). "Weight and hypertension: Evans County studies of blacks and whites." *Epidem. and Con. of Hypert.,* ed. O. Paul, pp. 177-205. New York: Stratton.

U.S. Senate hearing , Dec. 11, 1990, before Senate Committee On Labor And Human Resources on promotional practices in the pharmacutical industry.

Vogel, G., Trost, W., Braatz, R., et al. (1975) "Studies on pharmacodynamics, site and mechanism of action of silymarin, the antihepatotoxic principle from *Silybum marianum* (L.) Gaert. *Arzneim-Forsch.,* 25, pp. 179-185.

Wagner, H. (1981). "Plant constituents with antihepatotoxic activity" in Beal, J.L. & Reinhard, E. [eds.] *Nat. Prod. as Med. Agents.* Stuttgart: Hippokrates-Velag.

Waldholz, M. (1992). "New prostate drug from Merck wins FDA approval." *Wall St, J.,* June 23.

Walker, M. (1990). The Chelation Way. Garden City Park, N.Y.; Avery Publishing Groups, Inc.

Wallae, A.M. & grant, J.E. (1975). "Effect of zinc on adrogen metabolism in the human hyperplastic prostate." *Biochem. Soc. Trans.,* v. 3, pp. 651-655.

Watanabe, Y. (1982a) "Enzyme activity of hair follicles–especially with regart to glucose-6-phosphate dehydrogenase (G6PDH)." *J. of the Perf. Cos. Soc. of Jap. (pp. 9-414), v. 6, no. 1.*

Watson, R.R., et al. (1991). "Effect of b-carotene on lymphocyte subpopulation in the elderly humans: evidence for a dose-response relationship." *The Am. J. of Clin. Nutr.,* v. 53, no. 90-4.

Wattenberg, L. (1975). "Effects of dietary constituents on the metabolism of chemical carcinogens." Can. *Res.,* v. 35, pp. 3326-3331.

Weiss, R.F. (1988) "Herbal Medicine" *Ab Arcanum,* Gothenburg, Sweden, Beaconsfield Publishers LTD, Beaconsfield, England, p. 82.

Werbach, M.R. (1987). *Nutritional Influences on Illness,* pp. 211-212. Tarzana, CA: Third Line Press.

Werbach, M.R. (1988). *Nutritional Influences on Illness,* pp. 297-298. Tarzana, CA: Third Line Press.

Wical & Swope (1974). *J. of Prost. Den.,* v. 32, p. 13.

Williams, D.; 1993, "Public Service or Just Advertising Hype?", *Alternatives Newsltr.*

Williams, D.M., Lynch, R.E. & Cartwright, G.E. (1975). "Superoxide dismutase activity in copper-deficient swine." *Proc. of the Soc. for Exp. Bio. and Med.,* v. 149, pp. 534-536.

Williams, L.; "F.D.A. Steps Up Effort To Control Vitamin Claims", *N.Y. Times,* Aug. 2, 1992.

Wisniewska-Knypl, J., Sokal, J., Klimczak, J. *et al.* (1981). "Protective effect of methionine against vinyl chloride-mediated depression of non-protein sulfhydryls and cytochrome P-450." *Toxi. Letters,* v. 8, pp. 147-152.

Wolfe, Sidney; Health Letter, April 1993, Public Citizen Health Research Group.

Wynder, E.L. (1979). "Dietary habits and Cancer epidemiology." Cancer, supplement, v. 43. no. 5, pp. 155-1961.

INDEX